ABOUT THE AUTHOR

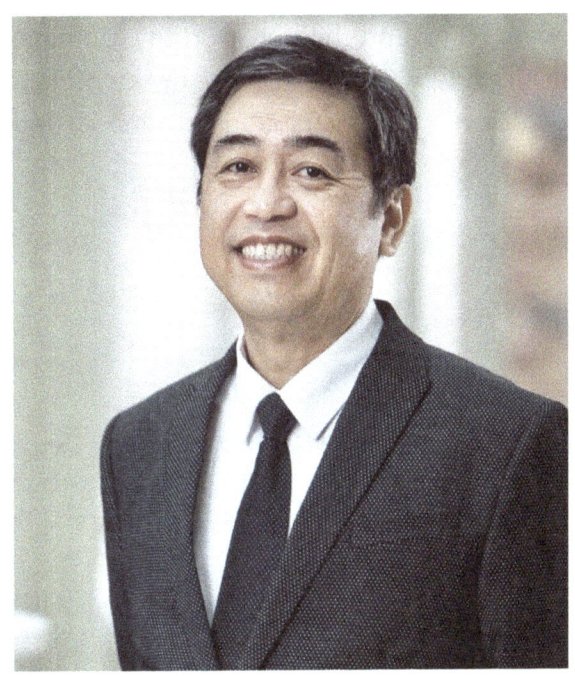

David Lardizabal, MD, MBA, FAAN., is an experienced academic and clinical neurologist. He was trained in Adult General Neurology in Cleveland Clinic Foundation, Ohio, and Philippine General Hospital. He was also trained in Internal Medicine at Cebu Velez General Hospital, Philippines. Dr. Lardizabal developed a passion for teaching clinical neurology with medical students during his residency training years and throughout his neurology career. He held academic positions at the University of Missouri, Columbia, Cleveland Clinic Lerner of Medicine, and Washington University School of Medicine in St. Louis. He has won awards in teaching and education innovation. He also advocates promoting value-based health care and improving public health policy.

ACKNOWLEDGMENT

I dedicate this book to my wife, Janet, and children, Dorothy, Dominic, Jaynell, and Joshua. They have been my inspiration in all my work. I acknowledge my mentors and patients who have taught me the art of neurological history, examination, diagnosis, and treatment.

Table of Contents

PREFACE	*4*
NEUROLOGICAL HISTORY SKILLS	*5*
NEUROLOGICAL EXAMINATION SKILLS	*8*
Types of Neurological Examination	*12*
Screening Neurological Examination	*16*
Common Motor-Coordination-Gait Examination	*24*
Deep Tendon Reflexes and Superficial Reflexes	*26*
Sensory Testing	*28*
Sample Problem Focused Neurological Examination	*29*
NEUROLOGICAL LOCALIZATION SKILLS	*30*
Neurological Disorder Category	*41*
Steps in Neurological Localization	*42*
LOCALIZATON CASES	*44*
DIFFERENTIAL DIAGNOSES	*50*
CLINICAL ASSESSMENT AND RECOMMENDATIONS (CARE)	*61*
Appendix I	*67*
Appendix II	*77*

PREFACE

This handbook is primarily intended for medical students. Medical students who start their education in neurology rotation are often challenged by the different neurological diseases and variations of neurological symptoms. Neurological diagnosis depends on a good history. The patients arrive with a story of their symptoms. The art of dissecting the patient's story and formulating a diagnosis and plan requires a systematic approach. The primary purpose of Basic Skills of Clinical Neurology is to help the student/learner construct a good interview, focus on pertinent examination findings, and logically arrive at a topographic diagnosis (neurological localization). This handbook *supplements* the students learning of neuroanatomy, neurological examination and neuropathology. After performing a neurological history and examination, the learner is taught the logical approach in organizing the neurological symptoms and signs. The principles of neurological localization and differential diagnosis will be presented in a simplified manner. This clinical skill is very fundamental in neurology. Without it, the learner will be lost in formulating the neurological disease's possible cause (differential diagnoses). Lastly, the student will learn to summarize the diagnosis and plan of care into a well-organized medical document.

NEUROLOGICAL HISTORY SKILLS

The gathering of neurological history is both a science and an art. An essential aspect in history taking is your listening skills, your empathy and showing interest in their problems. The patient and their family members are sensitive to your verbal and non-verbal (body language) communication. Hence, an excellent patient-physician rapport will facilitate the procurement of important medical information. The physician's bedside manners and communication are essential in gaining the patient's trust and increases their confidence.

The scientific part of neurological history taking is your skills and knowledge in neuroanatomy, neurophysiology, physical diagnosis, and neuropathology. The clinician will need a good background in internal medicine as many systemic diseases affect the nervous system. After a proper introduction, the patient's statement of the chief complaint will be the starting point in the History of Present Illness (HPI). The common complaints are headache, passing out, memory loss, language impairment, confusion, vision loss, double vision, dizziness, swallowing difficulties, focal or generalized weakness, fatigue, falls, imbalance, incontinence, sensory loss, tingling, involuntary movement, and convulsions. In the HPI, there are different ways of asking the patient of their chief complaint:

One is by saying "How may I help you?"

Another way of asking is: "What is bothering you?"

or "What is your main concern that made you primary doctor send you my way?

Some patients may not know why they were sent to a neurologist. Reviewing the referral sheet will help sort out the pertinent chief complaint. It is essential to be focused on the symptoms and not on the diagnosis given to the patient. Patients may have a misconception of their symptoms and wrongly attribute it to a specific disease. Some patients may tell the clinician that they are here for a second opinion of multiple sclerosis, seizures, or stroke. It is always good to be symptom-based in the chief complaint and history of present illness. This is to prevent biased questioning or preconditioning in the interview.

Patients do not readily give you relevant medical information in the clinic or hospital setting if you do not ask the right questions. Asking the right questions also indicate that you have a list of structures and diseases in mind. Like other medical specialties, neurologists are interested in the structures involved before making an etiological or differential diagnosis. Neurological disorders affect preferentially certain parts of the central or peripheral nervous system. Knowing the neuroanatomical involvement will help in the disease diagnosis as well as the differential diagnosis. It is important to remember that most neurological localization and differential diagnoses are usually formulated during the history taking. With these symptoms, one can perform the mental exercise of neurological localization. Arranging the symptoms in chronological order is important because it will help identify the proximity, progression, and relationship of the symptoms with the neurological structures involved. The temporal profile of each symptom is determined. Symptoms that occur within seconds or hours are often designated as hyper-acute. Symptoms less than a week are usually regarded as acute. Subacute conditions are symptoms less than a month. Symptoms of more than a month are considered chronic. For example, a patient with gradual memory and getting worse in 6 months is classified as a chronic progression. This same patient can also have a sudden generalized motor seizure after three months and the seizure is classified as a hyper-acute condition.

The temporal profile will also dictate the urgency of the neurological problem. An acute or hyper-acute presentation like fever, stiff neck, mental status changes, acute speech impairment, one-sided weakness, or ascending paralysis warrants more urgent evaluation and management. Neurological symptoms can repeatedly occur in a paroxysmal pattern, which is described as episodic. Some neurological symptoms may remain for days or weeks with resolution and may appear in another nervous system area after several months. This is often described as relapsing and remitting. Neurological symptoms that remain the same without improvement can be classified as static. Symptoms that continuously get worse without improvement are known as progressive. The impact of the neurological history on the daily activities or function of the patient should be considered. The basic activities of daily living include bathing, toileting, dressing, eating, and mobility. The social and emotional influence of the symptoms will give you a better understanding of the patient's condition.

Identifying risk factors in the past medical history, social history, and family history are essential in the diagnosis formulation. Patients whose history of present illness suggests a cerebrovascular disease (transient ischemic attack or stroke) may also reveal a history of coronary artery disease, peripheral vascular disease, hypertension, diabetes, and hyperlipidemia. The social history can adversely influence the occurrence and outcome of cerebrovascular diseases such as smoking, drug abuse, and alcohol abuse. In other neurological disorders, illegal drug use, tobacco use, recreational drug use, sexual habits, sexually transmitted disease, and home and occupational exposure (volatile agents, heavy metals, pesticides, carbon monoxide) may influence the current neurological problem. The family history is also helpful in evaluating the risk for epilepsy, vascular, neurodegenerative, neuromuscular, autoimmune diseases, and other genetic disorders. Some disorders are inherited like dystonia, epilepsy, Huntington's disease, and muscular dystrophy. Certain neurological disorders may not have a direct genetic linkage but having a family member may put the patient at a higher risk than the general population.

After the History of Present Illness is obtained, it is necessary to perform a useful review of systems. This will give an overview of the patient's overall health status. The review of systems should be based on symptoms that are active at least in the last 3 or 6 months. This may be time-consuming, but this will give the interviewer an insight into the patient's thought process and personality. It also allows the patient to relay symptoms that were not expressed in the initial part of the interview. Another vital component in the history is the medication history. It is crucial to list active and past medications. It is essential to be familiar with the dosages and side effects of medications. Dose-dependent side effects or idiosyncratic reactions that can have a contributing effect on the neurological problem. Figure 1 summarizes the general approach to neurological symptom analysis.

Figure 1. General Approach to Neurological Symptoms

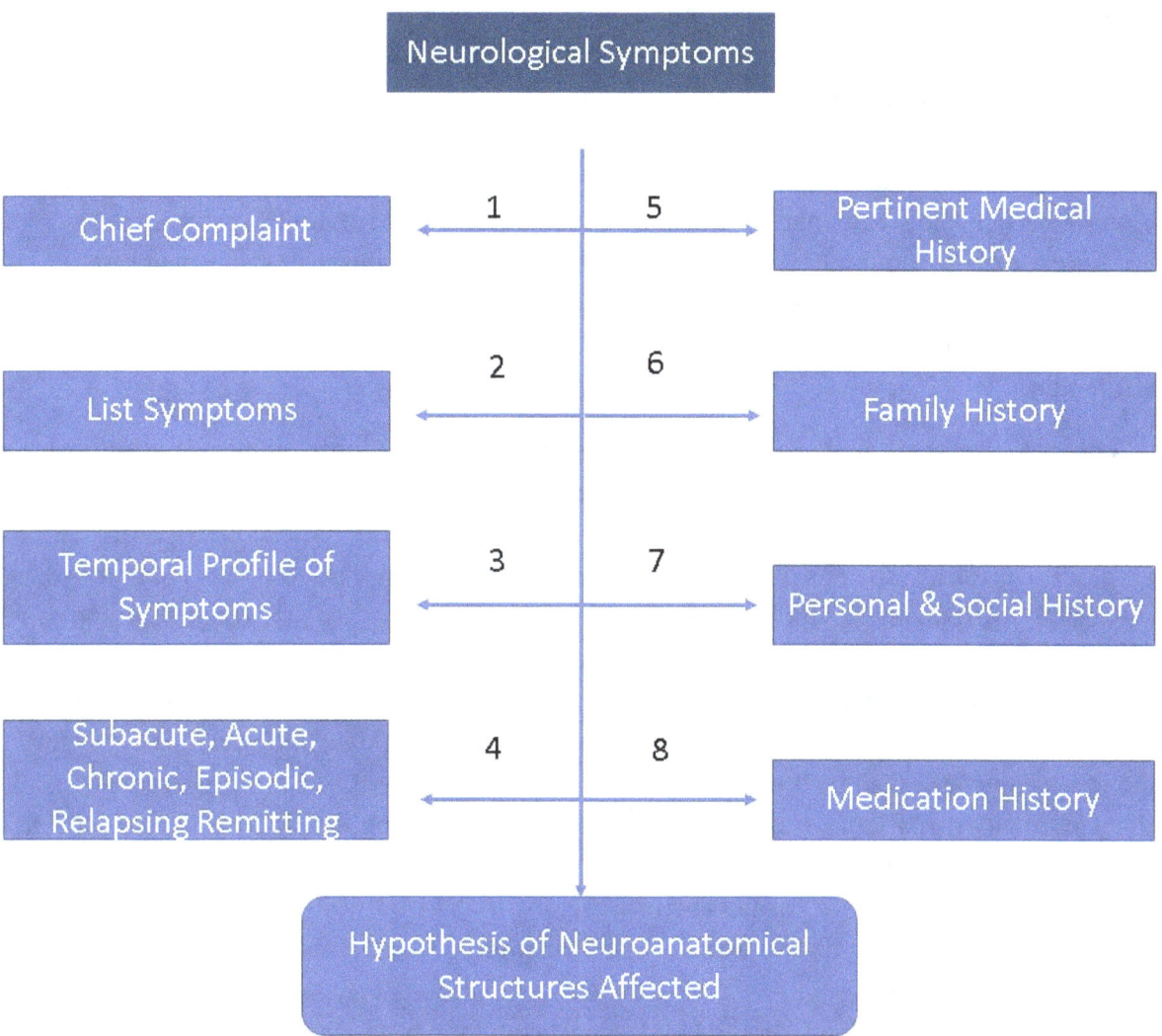

NEUROLOGICAL EXAMINATION SKILLS

The neurological examination is an integral part of the physical examination. Depending on the patient's clinical presentation, the neurological examination can be done early or in later part of the physical examination. There are three types of neurological examination: (1) Screening Neurological Examination, (2) Comprehensive Neurological Examination, and (3) Problem-Focused Neurological Examination (Figure 2). The clinician should have the necessary instruments in performing a comprehensive neurological examination (Appendix I). The neurological examination helps narrow down the structures involved by performing specific maneuvers that will elicit a loss or impairment of a neurological function. For example, the plantar response by stroking the sole will help determine if there is an upper motor neuron lesion (or corticospinal tract pathway lesion). An up-going big toe (Babinski sign) is characteristic of an upper motor neuron disorder. A plantar flexion response is a normal finding. Table 1 contains the list of common terminologies describing common neurological signs. These neurological findings are usually correlated with a neuroanatomical lesion or dysfunction.

A neurological screening examination will be enough in a wellness medical check-up with no neurological symptoms (Table 2). Often, neurological tools are not required but should be available if suspicious neurological findings were detected or if the patient has risk factors for a neurological disorder (such as diabetes). The mental status examination is focused on the alertness and responses to simple questions during history taking. The language function can be elicited by the patient's verbal fluency and auditory comprehension. The patient's reading and writing are also part of language testing. The patient should know their autobiographical information and be oriented to person, place, and time (month, day, and year). The memory functions can be assessed by the patient's ability to narrate recent and remote events. However, in elderly patients, the cognitive screening examination is evaluated in a structured fashion. The Mini-Mental State Examination (MMSE) by Folstein or using the Montreal Cognitive Assessment (MOCA) are useful in screening the mental status. The vital cranial nerves to screen are the visual fields and extra-ocular movements. This can be done quickly by confrontation testing and finger-following movements, respectively. Hypertensive and diabetic patients with a wellness check should have visual acuity and funduscopic examination as part of their general examination. Facial symmetry, hearing ability, articulation, and voice quality can be observed during the interview.

The motor examination screening involves facial strength, arm drift, finger tapping, finger to nose testing, hip flexion, ankle dorsiflexion, and heel to shin testing. The gait and balance are evaluated by the patient's regular walk and Romberg's test. The sensory test can screen for at least one primary sensory modality: light touch, pain, or temperature sensation of the face, arm, and legs on both sides. Light touch sensation is ideally performed with a wisp of cotton. The fingertips in light touch testing are not ideal but may be sufficient if you do not have the cotton or pin. Among people with diabetes, an internist usually screens for diabetic peripheral neuropathy using a monofilament. A screening examination does not typically check deep tendon reflexes or plantar responses unless there is a suspicion of a peripheral neuropathy or upper motor neuron disorder observed during the screening test. If a significant abnormality is found during the screening examination (such as spasticity), the clinician can decide to perform a problem-focused neurological examination or a comprehensive neurological examination (Figure 2).

A comprehensive or problem-focused neurological examination is appropriate when a patient has a single or multiple neurological symptom. A comprehensive neurological examination is essential during the patient's first clinical or hospital encounter (Table 3). This will establish the baseline clinical examination, which can be compared to succeeding examinations. The neurological examination tools needed are a penlight, ophthalmoscope, visual acuity card, sterile pins, tuning fork (128 Hz, 256 Hz/512 Hz), and reflex hammer. The mental status examination is like the screening neurological examination. But if the patient has cognitive problems, then a focused cognitive screening testing (Montreal Cognitive Assessment, http://www.mocatest.org/) or comprehensive mental status testing is performed. Table 4 outlines the different cognitive domains that are typically tested in a comprehensive mental status examination. If the clinician wants to have a measured and detailed cognitive assessment, a neuropsychological evaluation can be done. However, this is not typically done in clinics or hospitals. A neuropsychological evaluation is an elective test, and it may take a few hours to complete. Another type of problem-focused neurological examination is the NIH Stroke Scale. For example, a patient with an acute stroke and language impairment will need to be evaluated for the type of aphasia. The testing will include fluency, auditory comprehension, reading comprehension, repetition, naming, and writing. A combined comprehensive neurological examination and a focused neurological examination using the National Institute of Health (NIH) Stroke Scale can be used in a stroke patient.

The cranial nerve (CN) testing in a comprehensive examination covers cranial nerve I to XII (Table 5). The sequence in performing the cranial nerve examination may vary among clinicians. My preference is to start with the motor cranial nerves (III, IV, VI, V, VII, XI, XII) followed by the sensory cranial nerves (I, II, V, VII, VIII, IX) and cranial nerve reflexes. Pupil reflexes are mandatory in the comprehensive examination. However, smell (I), taste (VII, IX), corneal reflex (CN V, VII), gag reflex (CN IX, X) are not typically done unless there are symptoms directed to these respective cranial nerves. For example, if a patient has a loss of taste sensation, then smell testing is also needed. If the patient has swallowing difficulty, then gag reflex testing is mandatory. Primary sensory testing of the face may also be done during the sensory examination of the limbs and body. This is for convenience for the examiner so that the neurological tool used for the sensory testing (pin, cotton) are just used once. The cranial nerve reflexes II-III (pupil size, reflex), V-VII (corneal reflex), and IX-X (gag reflex) are done last for the convenience of the patient.

Moreover, corneal and gag reflex is also optional and should only be done if needed. In the written report, the cranial nerve findings are arranged accordingly from I to XII. Table 5 summarizes the cranial nerve testing procedures.

The motor examination should be systematic and attired appropriately (hospital gown, shorts, removal of footwear). The examiner should observe the muscle bulk and appreciate the muscle tone in all limbs. Motor power testing should evaluate proximal and distal muscle groups. Distal motor coordination should also be part of the testing. Station, gait, and Romberg testing can follow the motor examination. The superficial and deep tendon reflexes and primary and discriminatory sensory testing can be done in the latter part of the examination. The sequence of performing these tests also varies from one examiner to another. My preference is to test motor power, coordination, and gait in sequence. I perform the reflexes and sensory testing in sequence since it requires neurological tools. Test maneuvers that may be annoying for the patient can be done in the latter part of the test. However, this will also depend on the clinical presentation. Table 6, Table 7, and Table 8 summarizes the motor system examination, gait/station, reflexes, and sensory testing, respectively.

It is essential to learn that a comprehensive neurological examination should also be hypothesis-driven. The examiner has a hypothesis on which neurological domain is affected by the symptom. Though the comprehensive neurological examination covers most of the neurological examination techniques, the test's performance should be prioritized in which part of the nervous system should be tested first. Hence, if a patient complains of weakness, then it is logical to perform a comprehensive motor examination first and evaluate the rest of the neurological systems in the latter part. Students often think that performing the neurological examination should strictly follow the format of a neurological report. The neurology report is a standardized outline or summary of the neurological findings. Therefore, the neurological examination performance may vary because there are variations in the presentation of neurological symptoms. It will be a waste of effort if one thoroughly examines the cognitive functions (mental status examination) first when the presentation of the problem is acute low back pain and right foot drop. The clinician can proceed with a comprehensive examination of the back, the motor examination of the lower extremities, checking the deep tendon reflexes, and sensory testing of the lower extremities' specific dermatomes. The cognitive testing can come later, and screening MMSE may be sufficient.

During clinical follow-up, an experienced clinician does not need to repeat a comprehensive neurological examination to the same patient unless a change or progression of the disease or new symptoms has evolved. Once a physician has established the diagnosis (such as stroke), a problem-focused examination can follow the patient's neurological condition. A problem-focused examination can also be viewed as a syndrome-specific neurological examination (Table 9). The problem-focused examination's common goal is to make a quick assessment of the neurological disorder. An example of a problem-focused neurological examination is the National Institute of Health Stroke Scale (NIHSS). It is a neurologic examination that evaluates the effect of acute cerebral infarction on the levels of consciousness, language, neglect, visual-field loss, extraocular movement, motor strength, ataxia, dysarthria, and sensory loss. A single patient assessment takes less than 10 minutes to complete (see http://www.nihstrokescale.org/). Another example of a problem-focused neurological examination is the Brudzinski and Kernig's maneuver for meningitis. The resistance of passive neck flexion and knee flexion during the Brudzinski maneuver is indicative of meningeal irritation. The reader should review Table 9, which outlines the basic neurological test performed in different neurological conditions or diseases. With experience, a physician can develop their own set of problem-focused neurological testing. The use of neurological instruments will vary depending on the type of problem-focused examination. The learner can refer to Appendix I for the common neurological examination tools.

Figure 2. Types of Neurological Examination

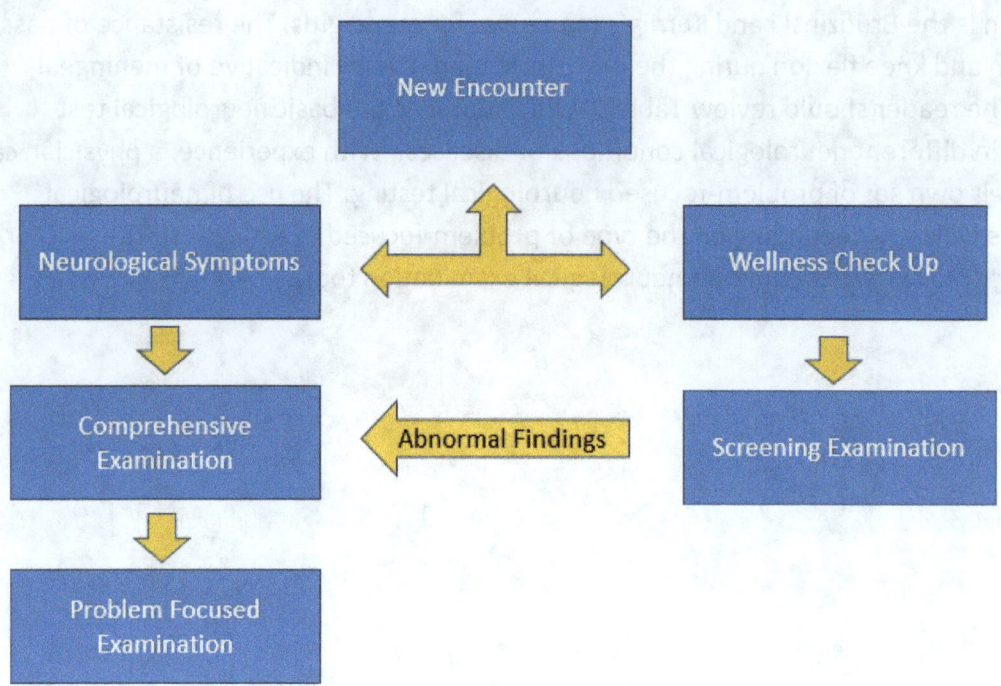

Table 1. Common Neurological Signs

Aphasia	Impaired language: this could affect expression, comprehension, reading, writing, or name.
Apraxia	Impaired skilled movement such as combing or dressing.
Hemi-Neglect	Impaired recognition on one side of the body, such as left hemineglect.
Acalculia	Impaired calculation of addition, subtraction, division, or multiplication.
Akinetic mutism	Inability to move and speak.
Agnosia	Inability to process sensory perception.
Astereognosis	Inability to process sensory input involving touch or feeling an object.
Auditory agnosia	Inability to process auditory perception. The person can hear the sound but cannot interpret the meaning of the sound.
Visual agnosia	Inability to process visual perception. The person can see the object but cannot interpret the meaning of the object.
Sensory Extinction	Impaired ability to perceive simultaneous stimulation of 2 analogous body parts. An example is sensory extinction of the left side of the upper arm when both arms are touch simultaneously with eyes closed. There is no significant loss of primary sensory modality on the side of extinction.
Visual Extinction	Impaired ability to perceive simultaneous confrontation testing of the left and right visual field. An example is left visual extinction when the two sides of the temporal visual field are tested simultaneously by the examiner. The patient has no visual loss when tested during the visual confrontation.
Anosmia	Inability to smell.

Nystagmus	Beating jerking movement of the eyes during primary gaze or gaze movements.
Opsoclonus	Fast, irregular, involuntary eye movements in different directions.
Strabismus	Impaired eye alignment.
Miosis	Small pupil
Mydriasis	Dilated pupil
Ptosis	Drooping of an eyelid
Eyelid Myokymia	Involuntary fasciculations of the eyelid.
Blepharospasm	Involuntary contraction of the muscles around the eye.
Facial Diplegia	Bilateral facial weakness
Dystonia	Involuntary sustained muscle contraction.
Spasticity	Increased muscle tone a limb that is velocity-dependent.
Rigidity	Increased muscle tone of a limb or body part that is not velocity dependent.
Babinski	An up-going movement of the big toe and fanning of the other toes during plantar stimulation.
Myerson's sign	Uncontrolled blinking upon repeated tapping of the above the nose and in between the eyebrows (glabella).
Hoffman sign	Flexion of the thumb upon flicking the terminal phalanx of the middle finger.
Tromner's sign	Flexion of the thumb and index finger upon flicking the volar portion of the middle finger's terminal phalanx.

Brudzinski sign	With the patient lying flat, there is the resistance of neck flexion accompanied by flexion of hips and knees.
Kernig's sign	With the patient lying flat, there is resistance on the extension of the leg when the ipsilateral hip is flexed.

Table 2. Screening Neurological Examination

Neurological Examination	Task performed
Mental Status Examination	Observe the level of consciousness and alertness
	Observe speech fluency, and comprehension
	Inquire about orientation to person, place, and date
Cranial Nerves	Visual Fields by confrontation testing
	Extraocular movements by finger following
Motor Examination - Strength and Coordination	Facial Strength - "smile."
	Pronated outstretched arms - checking for arm or pronator drift
	Finger tapping, Finger to Nose Testing
	Hip Flexion
	Ankle Dorsiflexion
	Heel to Shin Testing
Station, Gait, and Balance	Regular standing and walk
	Romberg's test
Sensory Testing	Light touch in both face, body, and limbs

Table 3. Comprehensive Neurological Examination

Neurological Examination	Task Performed
Mental Status	Observe consciousness, alertness, mood, and behavior
	Orientation to person, place, and time
	Verbal fluency, auditory/written comprehension, writing, naming
	Delayed and Immediate recall or 3 or 5 items
	Thought content, judgment, abstract thinking
Cranial Nerves (CN)	CN I Smell
	CN II Visual acuity, fundoscopy, visual fields
	CN II, III Pupil size and reflex
	III, IV, VI Extraocular movements
	CN V jaw opening and closure
	CN VII raising eyebrows, eye closure, smile
	CN VIII hearing rubbing of fingers near the ear*
	CN IX Observe swallowing movements
	CN X Palatal elevation by saying "Ah."
	CN XI Shoulder shrug and head-turning
	CN XII Tongue position at rest and on protrusion
	Test smell (CN I), corneal reflex (CN V-VII), taste (CN VII, IX), Weber's and Rinne's (CN VIII), Gag reflex (CN IX-X) if indicated.
Motor Examination	Bulk and evaluate the tone of upper and lower extremities
	Pronator drift of upper extremities
	Arm abduction, Elbow flexion/extension, Wrist Flexors
	Fine motor movements (finger tapping)
	Hip flexor
	Knee extensors, Knee Flexors
	Ankle dorsiflexors, plantar flexors
Motor Coordination	Finger to Nose testing
	Heel to Shin testing
Station and Gait	Standing, Romberg's test
	Tandem gait, Toe, and heel walking

Deep Tendon Reflexes	Biceps Reflex (C5-C6)
	Brachioradialis Reflex (C5-C6)
	Triceps Reflex (C7-C8)
	Knee Reflex (L2-L4)
	Ankle Reflex (S1-S2)
Superficial Reflex	Plantar Response (S1-S2)
Sensory testing	Light touch arms and legs
	Pinprick (or temperature) arms and legs
	Vibration of hands and feet
	Proprioception of fingers and toes

Table 4. Mental Status Examination

Consciousness	Normal	Abnormal
	Awake, Alert	Drowsy
		Stupor
		Coma
Language	**Normal**	**Abnormal**
	Fluent	Non-Fluent
	Intact auditory comprehension	Poor comprehension of auditory commands
	Intact written comprehension	Poor comprehension of written commands
	Intact object naming	Could not name objects
	Intact word repetition	Could not repeat words
	Intact writing	Unable to write
Calculation	**Normal**	**Abnormal**
	Could perform simple addition or subtraction	Unable to perform simple addition or subtraction
	Serial subtraction of 7 from 100	
Attention	**Normal**	**Abnormal**
	Could Spell WORLD forwards and backward	Could only spell WORLD forwards; Unable to spell WORLD backward
		Unable to spell WORLD forwards or backward
	Could perform serial subtractions by seven from 100	Unable to perform serial subtraction
Registration	**Normal**	**Abnormal**
	Could repeat three items immediately	Unable to repeat three items immediately
Digit Span	**Normal**	**Abnormal**
	Can perform 5 digits forward	Unable to perform 5 digits forward
	Can perform 3 digits backward	Unable to perform 3 digits backward
Delayed Recall	**Normal**	**Abnormal**
	Could recall 3 items after 5 minutes	Unable to recall 3 items after 5 minutes

Recent Memory	**Normal**	**Abnormal**
	Could recall events within the week	Unable to recall events within the week
Remote Memory	**Normal**	**Abnormal**
	Could recall remote events (birthdays, anniversaries, appointments)	Poor remote memory
Autobiographical Memory	**Normal**	**Abnormal**
	Remembers name, age, birthdate	Does not remember name
		Does not remember age
		Does not remember birth date
Visual-Spatial Task	**Normal**	**Abnormal**
	Intact Clock Drawing	Unable to draw Clock
		Hemineglect on Left side of Body
		Hemineglect on Right side of Body
Right Left Orientation	**Normal**	**Abnormal**
	Intact	Right-Left Confusion
Praxis	**Normal**	**Abnormal**
	Intact ideomotor praxis	Ideomotor apraxia
Gnosis	**Normal**	**Abnormal**
	Intact identification of objects by touch	Astereognosis
	Intact sound or word recognition	Auditory agnosia
	Intact visual identification of objects	Visual agnosia
	Intact finger recognition	Finger agnosia
Logic, judgment, and Abstraction	**Normal**	**Abnormal**
	Logical thinking	Unable to perform logical or abstract thinking
	Able to interpret proverbs	Unable to interpret proverbs
	Appropriate judgment of situations	Poor judgment
	Able to interpret similarities of objects	Unable to interpret similarities

Thought Content	Normal		Abnormal
	Lucid, coherent		Delusions
	No delusions or hallucinations		Hallucinations
	No paranoia		Paranoia
Mood and Affect	Normal		Abnormal
	Appropriate, Pleasant, Cooperative		Anxious
			Depressed
			Agitated
			Disinhibited, Impulsive
			Euphoric
			Manic

Table 5: Cranial Nerve Examination

Cranial Nerve	Normal	Abnormal
I	Normal	Abnormal
	Identifies smell in each nostril (use coffee, vanilla)	Cannot identify the smell (indicate side)
II	Normal	Abnormal
	Visual fields intact	Visual loss (indicate side)
	Distinct disc margins	Papilledema (indicate side)
	Disc to cup ratio < 0.5	Disc to cup ratio >0.5
	No narrowing of retinal arterioles; Retinal veins with intact pulsation	Absent retinal venous pulsation
		Retinal occlusion, narrowing
II, III	Normal	Abnormal
	Symmetrical pupils (indicate size, degree of illumination)	Asymmetrical pupils (indicate the size on each side)
	Direct and consensual pupil constriction is brisk	Afferent pupillary defect
III, IV, VI	Normal	Abnormal
	Primary gaze midline, full extraocular movements	Indicate side of eye and direction of weakness
		Ptosis
V	Normal	Abnormal
	Masseters and temporalis are symmetrical	Atrophy (indicate side and muscle)
	Jaw midline on opening and closure	Jaw deviation (indicate the direction of deviation)
	Symmetrical and intact sensation to light touch and pain	Decreased sensation to light touch or pain (indicate side and site)
VII	Normal	Abnormal
	Symmetrical facial movements upper and lower face	Weakness (indicate side and site)
	Can discriminate taste, anterior 2/3's of tongue	Absent taste sensation, anterior 2/3's of the tongue (indicate side)

	V, VII	Normal	Abnormal
		Brisk direct and consensual response to the corneal reflex of both eyes	Absent corneal reflex but can feel the touch of cotton (indicate side)
			Absent corneal reflex and cannot feel the touch of cotton (indicate side)
	VIII	Normal	Abnormal
		Can hear the whisper, finger rub, or ticking watch on each ear	Absent or decreased hearing (indicate side)
		Rinne's Test: Air Conduction (AC) > Bone Conduction (BC), Weber's Test (WT) vibration remain at the forehead	BC > AC, WT lateralized to the side of decreased hearing (conduction hearing loss)
			AC > BC, WT lateralized to the normal side of hearing (sensorineural hearing loss)
	IX, X	Normal	Abnormal
		Intact gag reflex bilateral	Absent gag reflex (indicate side)
	XI	Normal	Abnormal
		Can turn head towards the shoulder level, 5/5	Weakness in head and shoulder movements (indicate side, motor strength)
		Anteflexion and retroflexion of neck muscles, 5/5	
	XII	Normal	Abnormal
		Tongue midline at rest and protrusion	Tongue deviated on protrusion (indicate side)
		Symmetrical bulk, No atrophy	Atrophy, Fasciculation's (indicate side)

Table 6. Common Motor-Coordination-Gait Examination

Task	Nerve root	Nerve	Muscle
Upper Extremities			
Shoulder Abduction	C5/C6	Axillary	Deltoid
Elbow Flexion	C5/C6	Musculocutaneous	Biceps
Elbow Extension	C7	Radial	Triceps
Radial Wrist Extension	C6	Radial	Extensor Carpi Radialis
Finger Extension	C7	Posterior Interosseous	Extensor Digitorum Communis
Finger Flexion	C8	Anterior Interosseous and Ulnar	Flexor Digitorum Longus, Flexor Digitorum Profundus
Finger Abduction	T1	Ulnar and Median	First Dorsal Interosseous, Abductor Pollicis Brevis
Lower Extremities	**Nerve root**	**Nerve**	**Muscle**
Hip Flexion	L1/L2	Femoral	Iliopsoas
Hip Adduction	L2/L3	Obturator	Adductor Longus, Brevis, Magnus
Hip Abduction	L4/L5/S1	Superior Gluteal	Gluteus Medius/Minimus
Hip Extension	L5/S1	Sciatic	Gluteus Maximus
Knee Flexion	L5/S1/S2	Sciatic	Biceps Femoris, Semimembranosus, Semitendinosus
Knee Extension	L2/L3/L4	Femoral	Quadriceps
Ankle Dorsiflexion	L4/L5	Deep Peroneal	Tibialis Anterior
Ankle Inversion	L4/L5	Tibial	Tibialis Posterior
Ankle Eversion	L5/S1	Superficial Peroneal	Peronei
Ankle Plantar Flexion	S1/S2	Tibial	Soleus, Gastrocnemius

Coordination		Normal	Abnormal
Finger to Nose		finger to nose movements are smooth and coordinated	Dysmetria (indicate side)
Rapid Alternating Movements		Symmetrical, coordinated movements	Dysdiadochokinesia (indicate side)
Finger tapping		Symmetrical, coordinated movements	Slow or uncoordinated (indicated side)
Heel to Shin		Smooth, coordinated movements	Ataxic (indicated side)
Station/Gait		**Normal**	**Abnormal**
Standing up from the chair		Able to stand up from the chair without falling forwards or backward. It could be performed without using the armrest.	Unable to stand up from the chair. Fall backward during the attempt.
Casual Walking		Able to initiate walking and pacing well with balance. Arm swing and strides are coordinated. Turns are smooth without imbalance.	Describe if it is wide base, antalgic, spastic, myelopathic, steppage, ataxic, shuffling.
Tandem Walking		Able to walk heel to toe without imbalance or falling	Imbalance or tends to fall to one side.
Romberg's Test*		Able to stand upright with feet together with eyes open and closed.	Able to stand upright with feet together and eyes open; falls to one side when eyes are closed.

*Romberg test is a sensory test but usually done together with the station/gait examination.

Table 7. Deep Tendon Reflexes and Superficial Reflexes

Deep Tendon Reflexes	Neural Structures Involved
Jaw Jerk*	Cranial Nerve V Sensory (afferent)
	Cranial Nerve V Motor (efferent)
	Masseter muscle
Biceps Reflex	Cervical Nerve Root 5 (afferent)
	Cervical Nerve Root 6 (efferent)
	Biceps Muscle
Brachioradialis reflex	Cervical Nerve Root 5 (afferent)
	Cervical Nerve Root 6 (efferent)
	Brachioradialis muscle
Triceps reflex	Cervical Nerve Root 7 (afferent)
	Cervical Nerve Root 8 (efferent)
	Triceps muscle
Patellar Reflex	Lumbar Nerve Roots 2-4 (afferent)
	Lumbar Nerve Roots 2-4 (efferent)
	Quadriceps muscle
Achilles Reflex	Sacral Nerve Root 1 (afferent)
	Sacral Nerve Root 2 (efferent)
	Soleus/Gastrocnemius muscle
Hoffmann Reflex*	C8-T1 Nerve Root (afferent)
	C8-T1 Nerve Root (efferent)
	Flexor digitorum profundus muscle
Superficial Reflexes	
Abdominal Reflex**	Thoracic Nerve Roots 8-12
	Thoracic Nerve roots 8-12
	Rectus Abdominis muscle
Cremasteric Reflex**	Lumbar Nerve Roots 1-2 (afferent)
	Lumbar Nerve Roots 1-2 (efferent)
	Cremasteric muscle

Plantar Reflex	S1 Nerve Root (afferent)
	S2 Nerve Root (efferent)
	Flexor hallucis muscle (normal response); Extensor hallucis muscle (Babinski)
	Flexor digitorum longus (normal response)

*Optional; part in the screening of motor neuron disease.

**Optional; part in the screening of spinal cord injury.

Table 8. Sensory Testing

Primary Sensory Testing	Areas of Body Routinely Examined
Pain, Temperature, Touch	Face
	Distal and proximal limbs
	Peripheral nerve or dermatomal testing, if indicated
Discriminatory Sensory Testing	
Joint position sense	The distal joint of digit; the proximal joint is tested if distal joint sense is abnormal
Vibration sense	The distal bony prominence of the digit; proximal bony prominence if the distal bony bone is abnormal
Two-point discrimination*	Distal limbs, face, body, back

*optional; not routinely done in practice

Table 9. Sample Problem Focused Neurological Examination

Coma	Glasgow Coma Scale
Altered mental status	Language, attention, orientation, calculation, screening cranial, motor, sensory testing, reflexes, Brudzinski, Kernig
Double vision	Visual acuity, Visual Fields, Fundus exam, eye movements, pupil size, and reflexes
Headache	Head inspection, palpation, palpate temporal artery, temporo-mandibular region, evaluate Tinel's sign at the occipital region, neck movements, fundus exam, pupils, eye movements
Dizziness	Extraocular movements, Head Impulse Testing, Vestibular Ocular reflex, Limb coordination, Gait, Romberg's testing
Weakness	Eye movements, facial, neck, and tongue motor testing, limb motor power, muscle bulk, fasciculations, tone, motor power, deep tendon reflexes, plantar responses, sensory examination
Numbness	Detailed sensory testing head, body, and limbs
Back Pain	Spine inspection, palpation, straight leg raising test, manual motor testing, sensory, deep tendon reflexes, gait

NEUROLOGICAL LOCALIZATION SKILLS

Neurological localization is the synthesis of neurological history and examination to arrive at an anatomical or topographical diagnosis. It is a challenging mental task for medical students, neurology residents, and physicians. When I was a medical student, I was very impressed with my first mentor in neurology. After performing a focused history and neurological examination, he was confident in formulating the anatomical diagnosis. I was amazed that the imaging studies confirmed his neurological localization and diagnoses. During neurology residency training, I learned that a hypothesis-driven approach in neurological examination and localization was necessary for the anatomical and etiological diagnosis. My mentors required me to sketch the suspected lesion. I could only order a diagnostic test after I had defended the location of the neurological lesion. Without proper localization, unnecessary expensive procedures and treatment would occur. Novice clinicians are at risk of misinterpreting incidental findings seen in the brain or spinal cord. An astute physician should know the relevance of his clinical findings and correlate them with the diagnostic test results.

I still encounter students and neurology residents struggling in neurological localization. This chapter will show the step-by-step approach to neuroanatomical localization. Once you gain more experience, these guidelines will appear second nature or automatic. The basic knowledge of neuroanatomy and neurological examination is a prerequisite in understanding neurological localization. Hence, I advise the student to review the basics of neuroanatomy and neurological examination techniques. It is important to emphasize that neurological localization will be learned if one practices it periodically and consistently in patients with neurological disease. With practice, neurological localization becomes simple, intuitive, systematic, and organized.

Basics in Localization

Early learners in neurology try to localize the neurological lesion after the neurological history and examination. The mental process of anatomical localization and diagnosis is both dynamic and hypothesis-driven. The physician should start analyzing the symptoms with the chief complaint followed by the other neurological symptoms' sequence and progression. Questions and answers during the history taking and examination are probed to rule in or out the neurological structures involved in the disease process. Some parts of the nervous system have an eloquent and well-defined function. Hence, a neurological disease with a single lesion can manifest with a set of characteristic symptoms and signs (also known as a syndrome). Localization becomes more complicated if there are multiple lesions (metastasis) or specific portions of the nervous system (motor neurons, white matter). The initial approach in localization is to view the symptoms and signs from a broader perspective. One must look at the forest first before studying the trees. By logical deduction, the physician can narrow down on the specific area of the nervous system once he/she gathers more information from the history and examination.

There are different steps in localization. Each step progresses to a more detailed degree of localization. This logical approach should be made before arriving at the etiological and differential diagnosis. Each symptom or sign/s should be classified according to the Neurological Disorder and Division of the nervous system ([Figure 3](#)). This is conveniently called the "D's" of localization (Disorder and Division). Each symptom or sign/s should be categorized according to a Neuroanatomical Level, Lateralization, and Lesion type. These are also called the "L's" of localization. Finally, the neuroanatomical diagnosis should be formulated based on the overall correlation of the symptoms and signs. The steps of neurological localization are summarized in [Figure 4](#). The "D's" and "L's" of localization are described below.

Neurological Disorder:

Step 1: The first rule is to identify the functional group of the neurological symptom or signs. This can be deduced by grouping the signs and symptoms into a Neurological Disorder category ([Figure 3](#)). [Appendix II](#) contains the essential anatomical structures for each category. During history taking (or examination), arrange the significant symptoms (and signs) in chronological order. Try to group the systems which you logically think are related. It is also essential to note the temporal profile of each symptom because this will help in the differential diagnosis. The analysis starts with the chief complaint and with the other symptoms described by the patient. However, some symptoms and signs have no localizing value. The clinician should list the symptoms and signs that have a strong localizing value. Once the symptoms and signs are arranged, determine the neurological disorder category. There are ten neurological categories for neurological symptoms or signs:

1. Disorder of Consciousness

2. Disorder of Sleep

3. Disorder of Cognition, Behavior, Mood, and Thought Content

4. Disorder of Neuroendocrine

5. Disorder of Special Senses

6. Disorder of Brainstem or Cranial Nerves

7. Disorder of the Primary Motor System

8. Disorder of the Secondary Motor System

9. Disorder of Primary or Discriminatory Sensation

10. Disorder of Autonomics

By categorizing the symptoms and signs, the physician can focus more on what neurological structures are involved. Some neurological diseases may affect one or more neurological disorder categories. This first step aims to deduce the most likely functional group involved in the neurological disease. Anatomical correlation is facilitated by looking at this perspective. For clarification, Primary Motor System's Disorder indicates the pyramidal motor pathway (corticospinal and corticobulbar tracts) for the upper motor neurons and lower motor neuron pathways of the brainstem motor nuclei, alpha motor neurons of the spinal cord, and the peripheral motor nerves. For this book, the secondary motor system's disorder is the extrapyramidal motor pathways that centrally modulate the primary motor outflow. This usually involves the nuclei and pathways from the basal ganglia, brainstem, and cerebellum. The disorder of the brainstem and cranial nerves are grouped due to their proximity. Brainstem lesions may or may not involve their corresponding cranial nerves. Likewise, a corresponding brainstem lesion may or may not be present when there is a cranial nerve lesion. A detailed discussion on the anatomical structures for each neurological disorder is beyond the scope of this book. The learners are encouraged to read on neuroanatomy on each neurological category.

Neurological Division:

Step 2: After knowing the neurological category disorder, the next step is to determine the Division of the nervous system: Central Nervous System (CNS) or Peripheral Nervous System (PNS). The second step is essential because some neurological disorder categories can be a CNS or PNS problem; sometimes, it may be both. A combination of CNS and PNS usually indicates a systemic or disseminated disorder.

Neurological Level:

Step 3: The nervous system's level for each division should be identified for each symptom or sign. Each division has levels. In the CNS Division, these levels consist of the cerebrum, subcortical regions (thalamus, hypothalamus, pituitary gland, basal ganglia), cerebellum, brainstem, and spinal cord. In the PNS Division, these levels consist of nerve roots, ganglia, plexuses, cranial nerves, peripheral nerves (motor, sensory), neuromuscular junction, muscle, and sensory receptors. The cerebrum is the rostral level of the central nervous system. The spinal cord is the most caudal level of the central nervous system. In the peripheral nervous system, the most rostral and caudal levels are the nerve roots and sensory receptors, respectively.

The cerebral cortex (cerebrum) is mainly involved in higher cognitive functions like language, calculation, memory, visual and spatial orientation, music, behavior, and executive functions (abstract thinking, judgment, planning). The subcortical regions usually involve the basal ganglia, internal capsule, thalamus, hypothalamus, pituitary gland, which convey modulation of movement, endocrine functions, and reciprocal connections from the cerebral cortex, basal ganglia, thalamus, cerebellum, and brainstem. The brainstem level involves the midbrain, pons, medulla, and cranial nerves with motor, sensory or autonomic functions of the head and neck. The special senses are the structures involved in smell, vision, taste, and hearing. The special senses involve cranial nerves I, II, VII, VIII, brainstem, archicortex, temporal, parietal, and occipital cortex. The cerebellum is part of the secondary motor system and mainly controls balance, coordination, and muscle tone. The spinal cord has ascending and descending pathways involved in the primary motor and sensory pathways. In the PNS, the cervical and lumbar nerve roots and plexuses innervate the upper and lower limbs, respectively. Nerve root compressions or impairment attenuate the deep tendon reflexes and impair the specific myotome it innervates. It may also present with a dermatomal sensory loss. The brachial plexus and lumbar-sacral plexus pathology may affect the whole limb or partially the affected limb's sensory and motor functions. It has a broader spread of involvement than specific nerve roots or specific peripheral nerve of the limb. Peripheral nerve lesions may have pure motor, mixed motor-sensory impairment, and or pure sensory symptoms. The distribution may include distal and symmetric (stocking-glove distribution), asymmetric, or distributed in multiple body limb areas (multi-focal). Neuromuscular junction pathology may be localized (ocular, eye movements, eyelids) or generalized (diffuse). It does not have a sensory component. Muscle disorders typically affect the proximal and axial muscles earlier; however, there are muscle disorders that affect the distal limbs too. Small sensory nerve lesions may have symmetric, patchy, length-dependent, or length-independent distribution. Neurological level determination based on the chief complaint or history may be difficult to determine in some cases (undetermined). In these situations, the neurological examination will be necessary for defining the level, lateralization, and lesion type.

Neurological Lateralization:

Step 4. In this step, the clinician should decide which side of the nervous system is involved: left, right, midline (axial), bilateral/diffuse. There are distinct patterns of neurological symptoms or signs that can help the clinician deduce the lesion's side. If there are no lateralization features, then the pathology may be a diffuse or bilateral. There are specific patterns that are helpful in neurological lateralization:

A. In most right- and left-handed individuals, the left hemisphere is the dominant side for language. Hence, majority of patients with aphasia or dysphasia is lateralized towards the dominant hemisphere.

B. In the majority of right- and left-handed individuals, loss of visual-spatial orientation, and hemineglect is lateralized towards the right hemisphere.

C. CNS disorders of the cerebral hemispheres and brainstem have cross-symptoms. Hemisensory loss or hemiparesis is usually lateralized towards the opposite hemisphere. This is because the descending or ascending tracts of the central motor and sensory pathways decussate at the lower brainstem or spinal cord, respectively. When the lesion is below the brainstem, the central motor pathway involves the limbs ipsilateral to the lesion.

D. Intra-axial brainstem (within the brainstem) usually has crossed symptoms/signs of the ascending and descending pathways, and ipsilateral cranial nerve symptoms/signs. Extra-axial brainstem (outside the brainstem) lesions usually have ipsilateral cranial nerve symptoms early in the course of the neurological symptoms. Extra-axial brainstem lesions typically involve the descending or ascending tracts if the lesion has compressive or infiltrative effects.

E. Cerebellar hemisphere lesions are usually on the same side of the symptoms and signs. Midline cerebellar lesions affect the head and trunk (axial structures).

F. The lateralization of spinal cord lesions would vary depending on if the lesion is intra-axial or extra-axial and on the location of cord involvement (anterior, posterior, central, hemi-cord, or complete). The descending motor pathway would be ipsilateral to the side of the weakness. However, in ascending pathways, the primary sensory modalities like pain, temperature, and light touch deficits will be contralateral to the side of the spinal cord lesion. As for the posterior columns that carry proprioceptive and vibratory sensations, the deficits will be on the same side of the spinal cord lesion.

G. The lateralization of the motor/sensory roots (radiculopathies), plexopathies, and mononeuropathies are ipsilateral to the side of the symptoms and signs.

Neurological lateralization based on the chief complaint or history may be difficult to determine in some cases (undetermined). In these situations, the neurological examination will be necessary for defining the level, lateralization, and lesion type.

Below are examples of chief complaints that are localized based on Neurological Disorder, Division, Level, and Lateralization. After determining the Neurological Division, the *possible* level of the CNS or PNS involved should be cited in parenthesis. If Neurological Division may affect either or both CNS or PNS, then both divisions should be noted. Further queries in the history and neurological examination will help determine the correct neurological division. The lateralization should be cited as undetermined when the lateralization is not possible based on chief complaint or symptoms alone. In this case, the neurological examination will help refine the lateralization and lesion type.

Chief Complaint 1: I am becoming forgetful.

Neurological Disorder: Disorder of Cognition

Neurological Division: Central Nervous System (Cerebrum, Neocortex, Archicortex)

Neurological Lateralization: Possibly Left Hemisphere, If Right-Handed

Chief Complaint 2: I cannot feel my left face, left arm, and left leg.

Neurological Disorder: Primary Sensation

Neurological Division: Central Nervous System (Parietal Cortex, Subcortical/Thalamus)

Neurological Lateralization: Right Hemisphere

Chief complaint 3: I see double.

Neurological Disorder: Brainstem or Cranial Nerves

Neurological Division: Central Nervous System (midbrain, pons) or Peripheral Nervous System (CN III, IV, or VI)

Neurological Lateralization: Undetermined

Chief Complaint 4: I feel numb in both hands and feet.

Neurological Disorder: Primary Sensation

Neurological Division: Peripheral Nervous System (Nerve roots, Peripheral Nerves)

Neurological Lateralization: Diffuse or Bilateral

Chief Complaint 5: I cannot stand up from a chair.

Neurological Disorder: Primary or Secondary Motor System

Neurological Division: Central Nervous System or Peripheral Nervous System

Neurological Lateralization: Undetermined

Chief Complaint 6: I have tremors of both hands.

Neurological Disorder: Secondary Motor System

Neurological Division: Central Nervous System (Subcortical/Basal Ganglia, Cerebellum)

Neurological Lateralization: Bilateral

Chief Complaint 7: I have a spinning sensation.

Neurological Disorder: Brainstem or Cranial Nerves

Neurological Division: Central Nervous System (Brainstem, Medulla) or Peripheral Nervous System (CN VIII)

Neurological Lateralization: Undetermined, may be unilateral or bilateral

Chief Complaint 8: I keep on passing out.

Neurological Disorder: Autonomics

Neurological Division: Central Nervous System (brainstem, spinal cord) or Peripheral Nervous System (Peripheral Autonomic Nerves)

Neurological Lateralization: Diffuse

Chief Complaint 9: I cannot hear on my right side

Neurological Disorder: Special Senses

Neurological Division: Peripheral Nervous System (CN VIII)

Neurological Lateralization: Right

Chief Complaint 10: I feel electrical pain on the left side of the face

Neurological Disorder: Primary Sensation

Neurological Division: Central Nervous System (Parietal, Thalamus, Pons) or Peripheral Nervous System (CN V)

Neurological Lateralization: Right if CNS Division, Left side if PNS Division

Neurological Lesion:

Step 5: The type of neurological lesion is a topographical assessment of the lesion distribution in the nervous system. The clinician should correlate the neurological symptoms and signs and conclude if the lesion is in a single area (single lesion), multiple areas (multiple lesions), or diffusely in the nervous system (diffuse lesion). The operational definition of these lesion categories is explained below.

I. Single Lesion: the neurological symptoms and signs could be explained by a single lesion in a specific portion of the nervous system. There are two subtypes of a single lesion:

A. Focal Lesion: This is a discrete or point lesion in the nervous system. There is a specific point in the central or peripheral nervous system causing the symptoms and signs. A focal lesion has lateralizing findings (right or left). Examples of a focal lesion are root compressions (C6 or C7 radiculopathy), focal nerve entrapments (carpal tunnel syndrome and fibular nerve palsy), cranial nerve compression (vestibular schwannoma), cranial nerve inflammation (optic neuritis), and small ischemic infarct (lacunar stroke). A focal lesion has a minimal physical or metabolic effect (such as edema) on the surrounding neural structures.

B. Regional Lesion: This is a single lesion affecting a portion of the central or peripheral nervous system and has a more complex set of symptoms and signs. The neurological dysfunction from the single structural lesion is amplified by diaschisis, edema, a shift of the neuroaxis, or metabolic dysfunction. Regional localization is usually applied to lesions affecting the cerebral cortex due to its complex functions and connections. A regional lesion may have bilateral findings or lateralizing findings (right or left). In transcortical motor aphasia, the lesion occurs in the dominant frontal cortex region presenting with expressive aphasia, intact repetition, and comprehension. The etiology could be from vascular occlusion, hemorrhage, or tumor. Regional localization can also be found in the infratentorial region or spinal cord. A single lesion of the eight (VIII) cranial nerve from an acoustic schwannoma could be classified as a focal lesion if the symptoms and signs were isolated to unilateral hearing loss. However, an expanding acoustic schwannoma creates compressive effects in the region of the cerebellopontine angle leading to ipsilateral ataxia, dysphagia, and contralateral hemiparesis. In this case, the anatomical localization could be explained by a regional lesion in the cerebellopontine area. A metastatic compression fracture of the thoracic vertebrae can present either as a focal or regional lesion. If there was a single dermatomal sensory loss (T4), it is considered a focal lesion. If the compression fracture affected two or more contiguous cord segments and clinically manifest with a broad sensory level (T4 to T6 sensory loss), it is classified as a regional lesion.

The distinction of a focal or regional lesion may be problematic in the peripheral nervous system, especially in differentiating radiculopathies, plexopathies, and mononeuropathies. Radiculopathy and mononeuropathy usually indicate a focal lesion, but plexopathy shows a regional lesion.

The clinical distinction between a focal or regional lesion can be judged from the complexity of the symptoms or signs. As emphasized, a focal lesion is a point localization. However, a regional lesion can affect a specific point of the nervous system but have neighboring symptoms and signs due to the lesion's nature/pathology.

II. Multiple Lesions: the neurological symptoms and signs could be explained by at least two lesions that are in distinct parts of the nervous system. There are subtypes of multiple lesions:

A. Multi-Focal Lesions: These are multiple (at least 2) discrete or point lesions in the central or peripheral nervous system causing the symptoms and signs. Examples of multi-focal lesions are multiple sclerosis, multiple lacunar infarcts, and multi-focal motor neuropathy. The focal lesions have a minimal physical or metabolic effect (such as edema) on the surrounding neural structures. Multi-focal lesions should be *limited to 2 levels* of the nervous system (For example, cerebrum plus brainstem, cerebrum plus spinal cord, or brainstem plus spinal cord).

B. Multi-Regional Lesions: These are multiple lesions that have significant neighboring effects on the immediate surrounding neural structures. At least two regions of the central or peripheral nervous system are involved in causing the symptoms and signs. Examples of multi-regional lesions are metastatic disease to the brain, multiple parasitic infections, and embolic cortical strokes. Multi-regional lesions should be *limited to 2 levels* of the nervous system (For example, cerebrum plus brainstem, cerebrum plus spinal cord, or brainstem plus spinal cord).

C. Multi-Level Lesions: When there are *more than two focal or regional lesions* and *more than two levels* of the nervous system, the localization is classified as a multi-level lesion. Multi-level lesions have *lateralizing or focal neurological symptoms or signs*. Multiple lesions are considered multi-regional if the lesions are limited to 2 levels, i.e., cerebrum and brainstem. But if numerous lesions are distributed to the cerebrum, brainstem, and spinal cord, it is a multi-level lesion. For example, in metastatic disease to the CNS, it is multi-regional if only limited to 2 levels (cerebrum and brainstem). Once it disseminates to the cerebrum, brainstem, and spinal cord, it is a multi-level lesion from the metastatic disease. An essential feature of the multi-focal or regional lesion is that both have lateralizing symptoms or signs.

III. Diffuse Lesion: the neurological symptoms and signs could not be explained by single or multiple nervous system lesions. *There are no lateralizing symptoms or signs.* The central or peripheral nervous system involvement may be symmetrical or bilateral in distribution. Examples of a diffuse lesion are toxic-metabolic encephalopathy, acute disseminated encephalomyelitis, neurodegenerative disease, multiple system atrophy, and distal sensory polyneuropathy. The level of the neurological division involvement should be indicated when a diffuse process is involved. For example, diffuse encephalopathy means that the level of CNS involvement is the cerebrum or cerebral cortex. Diffuse white matter disease means that the subcortical area of the cerebrum is the level of CNS involvement.

Neuroanatomical Diagnosis:

The neuroanatomical diagnosis is the last step in neurological localization. The clinician should correlate the symptoms and signs with the neurological category, division of nervous system, level, lateralization, and type of neurological lesion. Each step in the symptom/s and sign/s should have a hypothetical anatomical diagnosis. The clinician can organize the symptoms and signs by constructing a localization flow chart ([Figure 5](#)).

1. The localization chart has multiple columns and rows. In the first column, the chief complaint and other symptoms are arranged in order. The chief neurological complaint is labeled as Symptom 1. Subsequent neurological symptoms should be labeled as Symptom 2 and so forth. The neurological symptoms that have clear anatomical correlation should be outlined.

2. Each symptom should be categorized in the subsequent columns. The second and third column is the Neurological Category Disorder and Division of the Nervous System, respectively. The fourth column is the Level and Lateralization of the Nervous System. The fourth column is the Neurological Lateralization. The fifth column is the Type of Lesion. The last column is the anatomic hypothesis for the symptom. Sometimes, the anatomical hypothesis may have more than one choice since the symptom can also be reproduced in another neural structural lesion.

3. Each abnormal neurological sign or abnormality in the neurological examination should also be arranged from the highest to least significance. The most significant abnormality is labeled Sign 1; the subsequent abnormalities are labeled as Sign 2, and so forth. Like Step 2, the clinician should categorize the neurological abnormality by the disorder category, division of the nervous system, lateralization, lesion type, and anatomical hypothesis. Sometimes, some related signs are grouped together. For example, right arm/leg spasticity, right hemiparesis, and right Babinski are signs related to upper motor neuron weakness. The anatomic hypothesis is a left corticospinal tract lesion.

4. After all the symptoms and signs are arranged, find a common denominator in the lateralization, lesion type, and anatomical diagnosis hypothesis in each row. The principle of parsimony may aid the clinician in the diagnosis. That is to formulate the simplest explanation for the constellation of signs and symptoms. In the localization summary, the clinician should attempt to make the provisional neuroanatomical diagnosis:

A. Single Lesion Neuroanatomic Diagnosis: If the lesion type in each row is a single lesion type and the anatomic hypothesis is concordant in each row, only one neuroanatomic diagnosis will be used. The neuroanatomic diagnosis should indicate the focal area or region of the nervous system.

B. Multiple Focal or Multi-Regional Neuroanatomic Diagnosis: If the lesion in each row is a multiple lesion type but limited to 2 levels and lateralizing features, a multi-focal or multi-regional neuroanatomic diagnosis will be used. The multi-focal or multi-regional diagnosis should indicate in order the anatomical structures involved.

C. Multi-Level Neuroanatomic Diagnosis: If the lesion in each row involves more than two levels, the distinct levels of the nervous system and lateralization should be indicated. For example, the right cerebral cortex, left brainstem, anterior spinal cord.

D. Diffuse Neuroanatomical Diagnosis: if the lesion in each row is the diffuse type, then the anatomical diagnosis should indicate the highest level involved in the diffuse process. The anatomical diagnosis should start with the word "diffuse," followed by the nervous system's highest level. Examples are diffuse encephalopathy (cortical/cerebral dysfunction) and diffuse symmetrical sensorimotor polyneuropathy.

Figure 3. Neurological Disorder Category

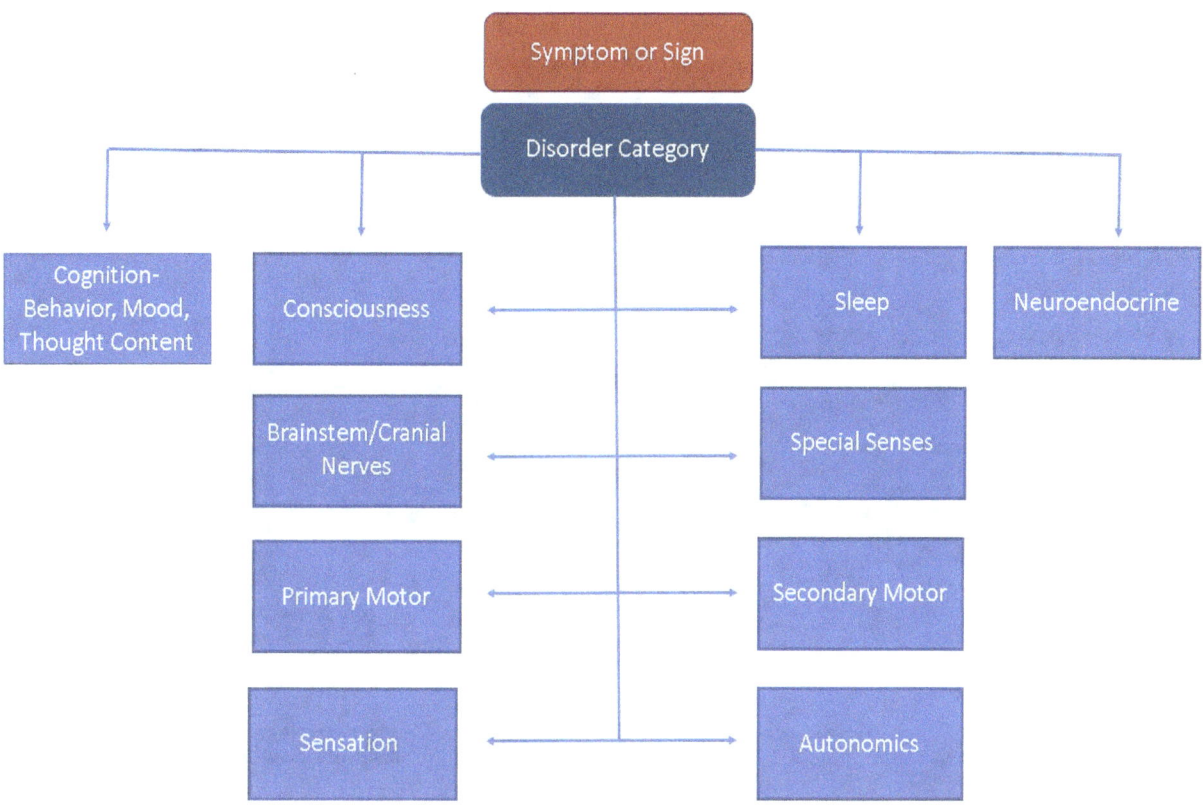

Figure 4. Steps in Neurological Localization

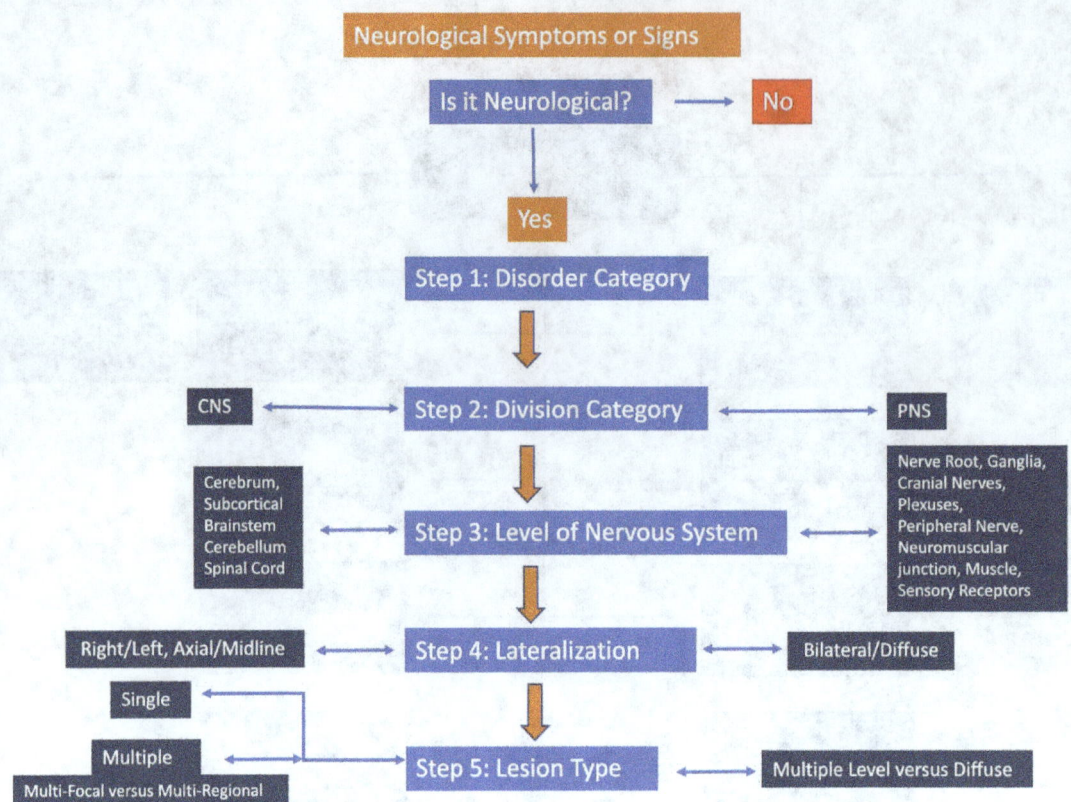

Figure 5. Flow Chart of Localization

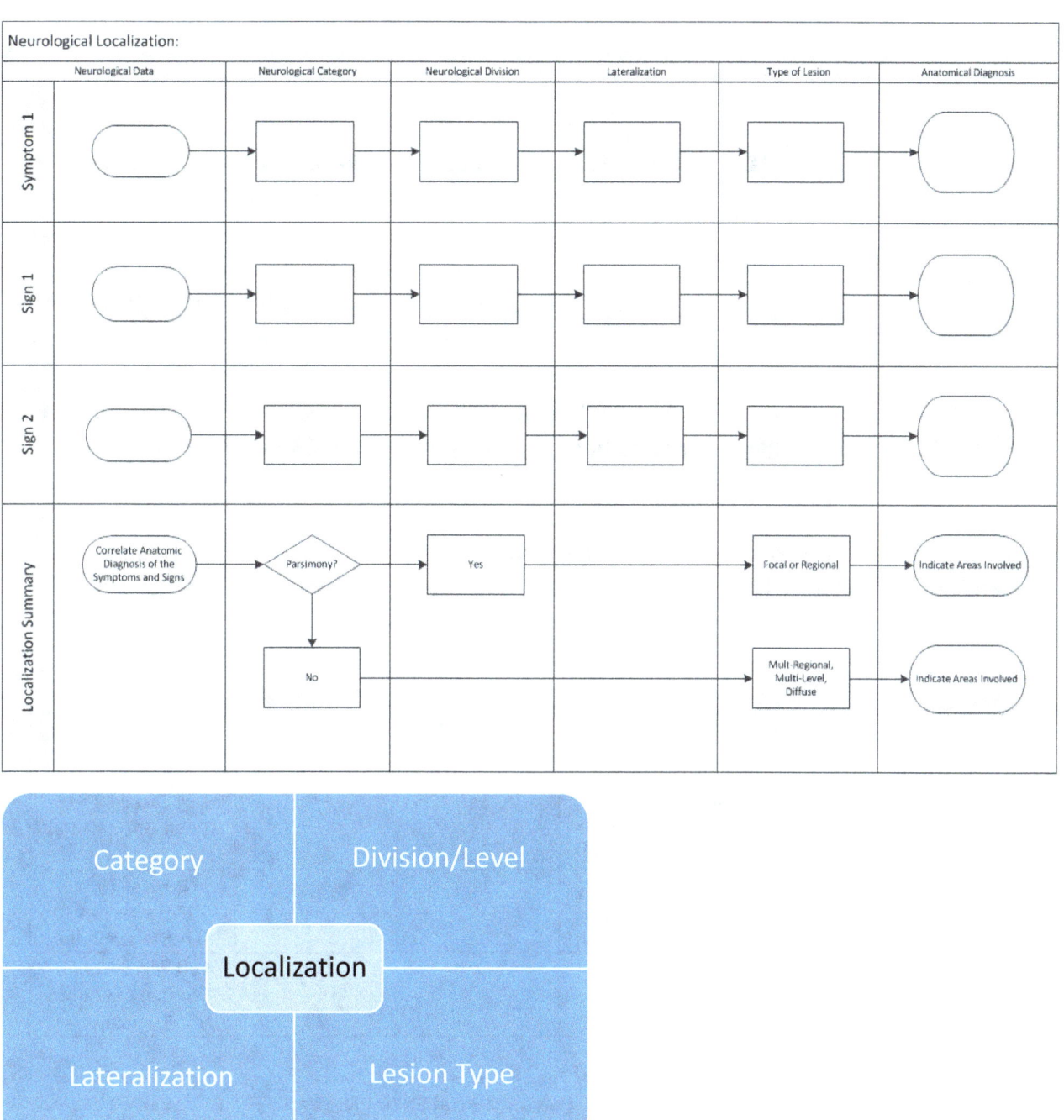

The flow chart of localization helps lead to a logical conclusion that correlates the salient symptoms and neurological findings (signs) with the anatomical structure/s.

LOCALIZATON CASES

Case 1.

AA is a 30-year-old female who experienced sudden pain behind the left ear. She discovered that the left side of her face was droopy. On examination, the head, eyes, ears, nose were normal. The mental status was normal. On cranial nerve examination, smell and vision were normal. The visual fields and optic disc were normal. Conjugate eye movements were normal. The jaw was midline on opening and closure. The face had a normal perception of light touch and pin sensation. The corneal reflex was normal. There was no wrinkling on the left side of the forehead when asked to raise the eyebrows. During forceful eye closure, the left eye remained open. The left side of the cheek did not move during smiling. There was decreased taste sensation on the left side of the anterior tongue. There was increased hearing on the left side. Palate movement and gag reflex were normal. There was a normal shoulder shrug. Head-turning was also normal. The tongue was midline at rest and protrusion. There was no atrophy or fasciculation. Motor power, tone, and coordination were normal. The deep tendon reflexes were 2/4 and symmetrical on the upper and lower limbs. The distal limbs had symmetrical perception to pinprick, light touch, and vibration perception. The joint position test was normal. The stance and gait were normal.

Symptom/Sign	Disorder	Division	Lateralization	Lesion Type	Anatomic Diagnosis
Facial Weakness	Cranial Nerves	PNS (Cranial Nerve, VII)	Left	Focal	Left Facial Nerve, CN VII, Facial Canal
Hyperacusis	Cranial Nerves	PNS (Cranial Nerve, VII)	Left	Focal	Left Facial Nerve, CN VII proximal to nerve to stapedius
Decreased Taste, anterior tongue	Special Senses (Taste)	PNS (Cranial Nerves, VII)	Left	Focal	Left Facial Nerve, Proximal to Chorda Tympani

Neuroanatomical Diagnosis: Focal Lesion, Left proximal Facial Nerve

Comment: The columns and row are all concordant that the neurological lesion belongs to the 7th cranial nerve on the left side. Specifically, it is a focal lesion of the left facial nerve.

Case 2

BB is a 55-year-old man with pain and progressive weakness of the left arm. The mental status testing showed normal speech and comprehension. He was oriented to person, place, month, and year. Recent and remote memory was normal. Cranial nerves II to XII were normal. On motor examination, the upper extremities showed a normal bulk and tone. The left-arm abduction was 4/5, and left elbow flexion was 4/5. The right arm showed normal strength. The lower extremities were normal. Coordination and gait were normal. Absent deep tendon reflex of the left biceps and other reflexes were normal in the upper and lower extremities. The plantar response was flexor. Sensory testing showed burning sensation and rash over the left thumb, left lateral forearm, left shoulder. There was a diminished pinprick in the same distribution of the left upper extremity. Pinprick, vibration, and proprioception were intact in the right arm and both lower extremities.

Symptom/Sign	Disorder	Division	Lateralization	Lesion Type	Anatomic Diagnosis
Decreased Arm Abduction	Primary Motor	PNS (Cervical Root, Peripheral Nerve, Muscle)	Left	Focal	C6 Motor Nerve Root, Axillary Nerve
Decrease Elbow Flexion	Primary Motor	PNS (Cervical Root, Peripheral Nerve)	Left	Focal	C6 Motor Nerve Root, Musculocutaneous Nerve
Absent Biceps Reflex	Primary Motor or Sensory	PNS (Cervical Root)	Left	Focal	C6 Motor Nerve Root
Burning Sensation of left thumb with rash, lateral forearm, left shoulder	Disorder of Sensation	PNS (Cervical Root)	Left	Focal	C6 Sensory Nerve Root

Neuroanatomical Diagnosis: Focal Lesion, Left C6 Nerve Root

Comment: The lesion is localized to the PNS on the left side. The lesion that could explain the neurological lesion is the converging point of the motor and sensory component of the C6 nerve root.

Case 3

CC is a 25-year-old male with neurofibromatosis. He developed hearing loss on the left side. For the last two years, the left extremities were clumsy. On examination, he cannot hear on the left side. The left face had decreased facial sensation on the left side. The right nasolabial fold was shallow when he talked or smiled. The furrowing of the forehead was symmetrical when he raised both eyebrows. Eye closure was symmetrical. He had difficulty targeting the examiner's finger on the finger to nose testing with his left hand, and heel knee to shin testing showed incoordination on the left lower extremity. The motor power was 5/5 and but increased tone of the right extremities. The gait showed slow pacing with the right leg. Finger tapping and foot-tapping were slower on the right side. He was unsteady with his right leg on tandem walking. The DTR reflex on the right upper and right lower extremities was brisk (3/4) with the extension of the right big toe with plantar stimulation. The left side DTR was 2/4 with a flexor plantar response. The sensory perception to pin, and light touch, and vibration testing were normal.

Symptom/Sign	Disorder	Division	Lateralization	Lesion Type	Anatomic Diagnosis
Left Hearing Loss	Special Senses	PNS (CN VIII)	Left	Focal	Cochlear Nerve, CN VIII, Left
Ataxia of Left upper arm and leg	Secondary Motor	CNS (Cerebellum)	Left	Regional	Cerebellar, Left
Right lower facial weakness, Increased tone and impaired fine motor on the right, Brisk reflexes of right Limbs, right Babinski sign	Primary Motor	CNS (Cerebrum, Subcortical, Brainstem, Pons)	Left	Regional	Corticospinal Tract, Left

Neuroanatomical Diagnosis:

Focal Lesion, Left CN VIII

Regional Lesion, Left Cerebellar Pontine

Comment: There is a focal lesion affecting the 8th cranial nerve. The 8th cranial nerve is situated on the left cerebellopontine angle. Due to the mass effect of the 8th cranial nerve lesion (such as a schwannoma), there is compression of the left pons, which affects the central motor pathways of the facial muscles and the descending corticospinal tract that control the right extremities. This would account for the upper motor neuron findings for the right side of the body.

Case 4

DD is a 45-year-old male with sudden onset of right-sided headache and loss of consciousness. The patient was unresponsive to auditory and noxious physical stimulation. There were sub-hyaloid hemorrhages on the right fundus. The right pupil was dilated, 7 mm, and nonreactive tonight (direct and consensual). The right eyelid was flaccid. The right eye was deviated to the right and down. There was no spontaneous movement. The plantar responses were flexor.

Symptom/Sign	Disorder	Division	Lateralization	Lesion Type	Anatomic Diagnosis
Sudden Right-Sided Headache	Sensation	PNS (Scalp, Skull, Meninges, Intracranial Vessels, CN V)	Right	Regional	Regional Intracranial Vessels (Circle of Willis)
Loss of Consciousness, Coma	Consciousness	CNS (Cerebrum, Upper Brainstem)	Bilateral	Diffuse	Both Cerebral Hemispheres or Upper Brainstem
Dilated, Non-Reactive, Right Pupil	Cranial Nerve	PNS (CN III)	Right	Focal	Right Oculomotor Nerve
Right Ptosis, Eye deviated right and down	Cranial Nerve	PNS (CN III)	Right	Focal	Right Oculomotor Nerve

Neuroanatomical Diagnosis:

1. Focal Lesion, Right Oculomotor Nerve
2. Diffuse Lesion, Upper Brainstem or Cerebral Hemispheres

Comment: New and sudden acute headaches usually indicate a vascular pathology (intracranial vessels, arterial or venous). This indicates widespread disruption of the critical structures related to consciousness (both cerebral hemispheres, upper brainstem) when associated with coma. The third nerve palsy could easily be localized by its characteristic findings (dilated unreactive pupil, ptosis, and eye deviation from the unopposed actions of the CN VI and IV). Ruptured cerebral aneurysms can present with both focal and diffuse localization findings.

Case 5

EE is a 57-year-old male complaining of pain radiating down the right anterior leg and difficulty walking. There were normal bulk and tone in the right leg; 3/5 strength in the right big toe extension and dorsiflexion in her right foot; 4/5 power in the right foot inverters and evertors. There were decreased pinprick and vibration sensations on the right foot's dorsum, including the big toe. The patellar and Achilles reflex was 2/4.

Data	Disorder	Division	Lateralization	Lesion Type	Anatomic Diagnosis
Radiating pain on the right anterior leg	Sensation	PNS (Root, Peripheral Nerve)	Right	Focal	L5 Sensory Nerve Root, Right
Decrease sensation to pinprick and vibration of the dorsum of the right foot and big toe	Sensation	PNS (Root, Peripheral Nerve)	Right	Focal	L5 Sensory Nerve Root, Right
Weakness of right foot dorsiflexion and inversion	Motor	PNS (L5 nerve, Deep peroneal nerve, Peroneal Extensor hallucis longus, Tibialis anterior, Tibialis posterior muscles	Right	Focal	L5 Motor Nerve Root or Deep Peroneal Nerve, right
Weakness of right foot eversion	Motor	PNS (L5, Superficial Peroneal Nerve, Peronei longus, and brevis muscle muscles)	Right	Foot	L5 Motor Nerve or Superficial Peroneal Nerve, Right

Neuroanatomical Diagnosis: Focal Lesion, Right L5 Nerve Root

Comment: Acute back pain and radiating pain to the lower extremities usually indicate a nerve root entrapment. When it affects a single root, it has a characteristic myotome and sensory dermatome distribution. In this case, the L5 nerve root involved mainly the myotomes responsible for ankle dorsiflexion, eversion, and inversion of the foot. The sensory dermatomal involvement was demonstrated with the loss of the primary sensory modalities of the dorsum of the foot and big toe. Moreover, the distribution of the shooting pain can also give a clue to the sensory dermatome involved. There is no deep tendon reflex testing that can localize L5 nerve root lesions. Nevertheless, it helped exclude L2-L3-L4 and S1-S2 nerve root lesions. S1 radiculopathy may show a depressed or absent ankle jerk (S1-S2).

Case 6

FF is a 72-year-old female with a 10-month history of progressive gait difficulty, right leg numbness, and urinary incontinence. The mental status examination was normal. Cranial nerves testing II to XII were normal. The motor examination of the upper extremities showed normal bulk and tone and 5/5 power. On the lower extremities, there was normal bulk. The muscle tone was increased on the left leg with 5/5 strength except for the left hip flexion, 4/5. The deep tendon reflexes were 2/4 except for the left knee 4/4 and left ankle 4/4. There was positive ankle clonus on the left foot. The coordination and showed normal finger to nose testing and heel to knee to shin testing. The patient demonstrated an unsteady gait and stiff legs during walking. On sensory testing, decrease pinprick perception on the right side (lower abdomen, right leg) side just below the umbilicus; vibration and proprioception perception was reduced in the left foot and leg. All other sensation was intact.

Data	Disorder	Division	Lateralization	Lesion Type	Anatomic Diagnosis
Difficulty in walking	Primary or Secondary Motor	CNS, PNS	Undetermined	Undetermined	Undetermined
Left Hip Flexion, Weakness, Left Leg Hypertonia, Left 4/4 Patellar, 4/4 Achilles DTR	Primary Motor	CNS (Spinal Cord)	Left	Focal, Regional	Left anterolateral spinal cord (thoracic or Lumbar)
Diminished pain sensation on the right side below the umbilicus	Sensation	CNS	Left	Focal or Regional	Left anterolateral spinal cord (T10)
Decreased proprioception, vibration left lower leg	Sensation	CNS	Left	Focal, Regional	Left posterior spinal cord (thoracic or lumbar)

Neuroanatomical Diagnosis: Regional Lesion, Left Hemicord, T10 level

Comment: There is a combination of primary motor and primary sensory disturbance. The presence of a sensory demarcation just below the umbilicus on the right side provided the level of the lesion. In this case, the T10 spinal cord level. The diminished vibration sense and upper motor neuron findings on the left lower extremity lateralized the lesion towards the spinal cord's left side. The corticospinal tract and spinothalamic tracts on the spinal cord are anterior lateral in location. Proprioceptive functions are posterior cord in location. Hence, the left side of the T10 spinal cord is the site of the lesion. It is a regional type of lesion since it affects the cord's whole left side at the T10 level.

DIFFERENTIAL DIAGNOSES

It is essential to generate a hypothesis on the clinical diagnoses for each patient. This hypothesis leads to the formulation of the differential diagnoses where a list of diseases is grouped based on similar clinical, laboratory, and imaging features. It is the art of distinguishing these similar diseases from one another and coming up with the most likely diagnosis. It is a personalized or tailored list for a specific patient. The differential diagnoses require an excellent integration of history, examination, localization, disease progression, and pathology/disease mechanism. These are basic skill sets that a physician must learn in differential diagnosis formulation. These steps are outlined in this chapter.

Step 1: Illness Script:

The patient's illness script summarizes the relevant points in the history, examination, and neurological localization. The first sentence should be the salient symptoms along with the temporal profile of the most important symptom. The next sentence should contain the salient signs in the clinical examination. The data from the historical symptoms and clinical findings are the same in the clinical localization chart. The additional item in the patient script is the temporal profile of the symptoms. The symptoms could be acute, progressive, or chronic. The third sentence is usually the clinical localization of the patient script.

Example of a Patient's Illness Script:

A.B. is a 24-year-old female who developed an acute severe headache and bilateral blindness in her third trimester of pregnancy. There was no light perception for both eyes. The pupils were symmetrically dilated and unreactive. There was neck stiffness on head flexion. Extraocular movements were normal. The rest of the cranial nerves, motor, sensory examination was normal. The neurological deficit is localized to the optic chiasm. The neck stiffness suggests a diffuse meningeal involvement.

Step 2: Patient's Disease Syndrome Script:

Clinical experts learn how to recognize the salient symptoms and signs for a group of diseases. A group of neurological disorders tends to affect areas of the nervous systems and present with similar symptoms and signs.

These groups of similar symptoms and signs are often described as neurological syndromes (syndrome diagnoses). Hence, a neurological syndrome may contain three or more specific neurological diseases. A descriptive summary of each *neurological syndrome* is called a *Disease*

Syndrome Script. A clinician needs to match the patient's clinical features with a neurological disease syndrome. Below are examples of neurological syndromes:

Dementia: the gradual or rapid loss of 2 or more cognitive functions like memory, speech, visual-spatial functions, executive planning, and orientation. A co-morbid psychiatric disorder often accompanies it.

Stroke: acute onset neurological deficit that can be attributed to a specific vascular territory.

Parkinsonism: a gradual neurological disorder associated with rigidity, tremors, gait disturbance, and imbalance.

Epilepsy: the recurrent risk of having focal or generalized seizures. The clinical presentation would vary depending on the site of the seizure was generated.

Bell's Palsy: an acute unilateral weakness of the facial muscles.

Myelopathy: an acute or chronic dysfunction of the spinal cord causing upper motor neuron weakness of all four limbs or lower limbs associated with sensory disturbance or bladder/bowel dysfunction.

Myopathy: an acute or chronic dysfunction of the muscles causing lower motor neuron weakness or cramping. It typically involves the proximal limbs. There are no sensory symptoms.

Polyneuropathy: an acute or chronic dysfunction of the motor, sensory or mixed motor-sensory peripheral nerves of the limbs. It is usually length-dependent and affects the distal limbs.

Myasthenia Syndrome: a chronic dysfunction of the neuromuscular junction manifested as exertional weakness of the bulbar or limb muscles. There are no sensory symptoms.

Patient Disease Syndrome Example:

A.B. is a 24-year-old female in her third trimester of pregnancy who presents with an acute severe headache and bilateral blindness. There was no light perception for both eyes. The pupils were dilated and unreactive pupils. There was neck stiffness on head flexion. Extraocular movements were normal. The rest of the cranial nerves, motor, sensory examination was normal. This is consistent with an optic cranial neuropathy syndrome localized to the optic chiasm. The acute headache syndrome has no localizing features but suggests a diffuse meningeal involvement.

Step 3: Patient's Disease Script

A descriptive summary of a specific *neurological disease* is called a *Disease Script*. Figure 6 illustrates the essential details incorporated in a Disease Script. It contains the clinical localization, salient symptoms and signs (syndrome), epidemiology, temporal profile, and disease mechanism (pathology). The important feature of the patient disease script is the *disease category mechanism*, as discussed below.

Neurological Disease Mechanism/Category:

There are mnemonics to remember the different neurological disease mechanisms. The most frequently used mnemonic is the VITAMIN CDE (as outlined below). In selecting the various neurological disease mechanisms, the temporal profile of the symptoms will be relevant in the selection. If the disease mechanism is unknown, it would be cited as unknown (U).

Neurological Disease Mechanism	Temporal Profile
VASCULAR (V)	Acute > Chronic
INFLAMMATORY/INFECTIOUS (I)	Acute > Subacute > Chronic
TRAUMATIC/TOXIC (T)	Acute > Subacute
AUTOIMMUNE (A)	Subacute > Chronic
METABOLIC (M)	Acute > Subacute
IATROGENIC (I)	Acute > Subacute > Chronic
NEOPLASTIC (N)	Chronic > Subacute
CONGENITAL (C)	Chronic
DEGENERATIVE (D)	Chronic
ENDOCRINE (E)	Chronic > Subacute > Acute

Vascular Category:

Vascular neurological events are usually sudden (acute or hyper-acute) and occurring within seconds or minutes. It may be ischemic or hemorrhagic. Ischemic events may be arterial or venous. Arterial ischemic lesions produce acute stroke syndromes such as lacunar strokes or large vessel occlusion. These ischemic stroke syndromes have been well described in neurology textbooks. The reader is advised read more on classic ischemic stroke syndromes in general neurology textbooks. Venous (or venous sinus) ischemic strokes are not as common with arterial strokes. Hemorrhagic lesions may be intraparenchymal, subarachnoid, subdural, or intraventricular. Depending on the vascular lesion's location and extent, the symptoms and signs may have focal, multifocal, multi-regional, or diffuse localization. Non-parenchymal hemorrhagic lesions (subarachnoid, epidural, subdural, intraventricular) usually present with non-localizing signs (confusion, headaches). Chronic vascular events are commonly seen with subdural hematomas, which may have started acutely but with mild neurological symptoms. The mass effect of the subdural hematoma creates multi-regional or multi-level neurological symptoms.

Inflammatory or Infectious Category:

The inflammatory neurological category usually indicates an infectious cause. They typically present with some acute symptoms if the offending organisms are bacterial or viral. Fungal, parasitic, mycobacterial, or prion diseases usually present with a chronic course.

Traumatic or Toxic Category:

Traumatic injuries are acute and can affect the CNS, PNS, or both. The injuries may be penetrating or non-penetrating. Toxicological causes for neurological diseases may be acute or subacute in presentation. An exogenous substance that is absorbed, inhaled, or ingested is usually heavy metals, chemotherapy drugs, or prescription medications. Acute or long-term exposure to pollutants or gases may also lead to neurological disorders.

Autoimmune Category:

The immune system can affect different CNS and PNS levels (brain, peripheral nerves, neuromuscular junction, muscles). Systemic autoimmune diseases may also involve the intracranial and extracranial vasculature or multiple organs (thyroid, lungs, kidneys, and skin). Common systemic autoimmune diseases include Systemic Lupus Erythematosus and Sjogren's diseases. A classic example of neurological autoimmune disease is Myasthenia Gravis. Acetylcholine receptor autoantibodies interfere with post-synaptic neuromuscular junction transmission. Remote effects of malignancies outside the nervous system are also known as Paraneoplastic Syndrome. Lung, breast, and ovarian malignancies are common primary malignancies that can cause a paraneoplastic syndrome to the CNS, PNS, or both.

Metabolic Category:

Metabolic disorders affecting the CNS or PNS usually indicate an endogenous derangement of the human physiology that is not caused by environmental exposure or ingestion of a toxic substance. Electrolyte imbalance such as hypo-or hypernatremia, hypo-or hyperkalemia, hypo-or hypercalcemia, hypo-or hypermagnesemia can cause a diffuse effect on the CNS or PNS. Sodium imbalance commonly led to diffuse cerebral dysfunction or encephalopathy. Potassium imbalance typically led to muscle weakness or myopathy. Calcium and magnesium imbalance can cause both CNS or PNS dysfunction. Organ failure of the kidney and liver is another source of metabolic dysfunction affecting the CNS or PNS disease. Liver failure from liver cirrhosis causes an accumulation of ammonia and hepatic encephalopathy. Acute or chronic renal failure has a similar clinical presentation with liver failure. Acute or chronic diffuse dysfunction of the cerebral hemispheres will lead to poor attention, disorientation, and alteration of the level of awareness/consciousness. There are also metabolic disorders that are predominantly from an underlying genetic condition. Hence, metabolic and genetic causes of neurological disorders may overlap.

Iatrogenic Category:

Iatrogenic causes of neurological diseases are inadvertent consequences from a diagnostic procedure or treatment. Invasive diagnostic procedures (needle aspiration, endoscopy, surgical biopsies) may lead to bleeding or infection. Interventional radiological procedures (angiogram) may cause contrast adverse effects or vascular dissection. There are some adverse reactions to medical treatment. Idiosyncratic drug reactions from anti-seizure drugs may cause CNS toxicity (encephalopathy, dizziness, imbalance, nystagmus) even at standard dosages. Anaphylactic drug reactions like cutaneous drug eruptions may also occur during treatment. Radiation treatment of brain tumors may have delayed effects on the CNS, causing radiation-related necrosis, edema, and white matter changes.

Neoplastic Category:

Primary benign tumors, malignant tumors, or metastatic tumors can affect the CNS and PNS from their direct mechanical/infiltrative effects. Edema surrounding a primary or metastatic tumor will produce more profound symptoms to neighboring areas (diaschisis). Metastatic diseases can also affect the vasculature of CNS, i.e., intravascular lymphomas or circulation of the cerebrospinal fluid, i.e., leptomeningeal carcinomatosis.

Congenital Category:

Congenital disorders of the nervous system are diseases that occur in utero. This may be from an underlying genetic disorder, exposure to a drug/toxin, or infection of the CNS in utero. Congenital brain anomalies may be from malformation or disruption of brain development.

Malformations of brain development (anencephaly, cortical dysplasia) may be from an inherent genetic disorder or spontaneous somatic mutation. Disruption of brain development is caused by environmental exposure (toxins, infection, radiation) that interferes with neurons' proliferation and migration. It can lead to acquired genetic or secondary genetic mutations of brain development. TORCH infections (Toxoplasma, Rubella, Cytomegalovirus, Herpes Simplex Virus), chemical, radiation exposure, intrauterine hypoxia are common causes of congenital brain developmental disorders. Recently, infection with the Zika virus from mosquitos can lead to anencephaly.

Degenerative Category:

Neurodegenerative diseases commonly involve the adults or elderly age group. In the CNS, the common neurodegenerative disorders predominantly affect higher mental faculties or motor functions. There are two main categories of neurodegenerative brain disorders, Tauopathy and Synucelinopahty. Abnormal accumulation of tau proteins in brain cells can lead senile dementia, progressive supranuclear palsy, corticobasal degeneration, and frontotemporal dementia. The tauopathies may predominantly affect higher cognitive functions. Alzheimer's Disease (AD) and Fronto-Temporal Dementia (FTD) are common neurodegenerative brain diseases that affect cognition and memory. Among the synucleinopathies, Parkinson's disease is the most common disorder. An abnormal synuclein aggregation (Lewy bodies) leads to dopaminergic cells' death and Parkinson's disease. Other neurodegenerative diseases may affect a specific set of neurons. Amyotrophic Lateral Sclerosis predominantly affects the motor neurons of the brain and spinal cord. In Parkinson's disease and ALS, cognitive or psychiatric symptoms may occur as the disease progresses.

Endocrine Category:

Neuroendocrine disorders are disorders that affect the hypothalamic-pituitary functions. Pituitary tumors may have an overproduction or underproduction of a specific hormone. An example would be a prolactin-secreting pituitary tumor. Growth hormone over-secretion may lead to gigantism. Some endocrine organs outside the CNS, like the thyroid and adrenal glands, can also cause neurological symptoms. Hypothyroidism can cause headaches and cognitive impairment. Diabetes Mellitus is a common endocrine disorder that also causes peripheral neuropathy.

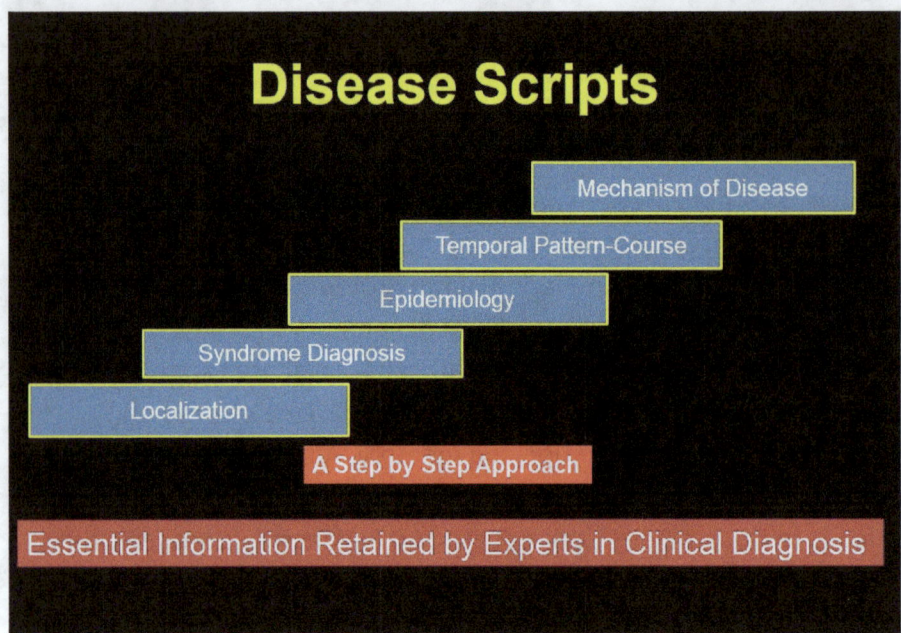

Figure 6. Disease Scripts

With experience, the physician would remember the epidemiology, disease mechanism, and temporal course. It is easier to remember the different disease mechanisms by their neurological disease category. Specific disease mechanisms have a typical temporal profile.

Patient Disease Script Example:

A.B. is a 24-year-old female who presents with an acute severe headache and bilateral blindness in her third trimester of pregnancy. There was no light perception for both eyes. The pupils were dilated and unreactive. The neck was neck stiffness on head flexion. Extraocular movements were normal. The rest of the cranial nerves, motor, sensory examination was normal. This is consistent with an acute headache syndrome with possible diffuse meningeal involvement and acute optic nerve cranial neuropathy syndrome affecting the optic chiasm (integration of Steps 1 and 2). This is likely from a vascular or inflammatory disease pathology (Step 3).

As we gain more clinical experience, patient illness script and disease syndrome formulation become very straightforward. An experienced clinician can directly formulate the Disease Script and skip steps 1 and 2.

Step 4: Diagnostic Triad:

Since many neurological diseases may belong to a specific syndrome, the physician should prioritize the top 3 diseases based on the clinical history, examination, localization, temporal profile, epidemiology, and disease mechanism (Step 1 to 3). In Figure 7, the patient disease scripts have three diagnoses (diagnosis A, B, C) that overlap. The three diagnoses are known as the Diagnostic Triad of the patient's disease syndrome. The diagnostic triad may belong to one or more neurological disease categories, i.e., infectious or autoimmune. In the diagnostic triad, the diagnoses are tiered or prioritized according to the level of probability of diagnosis:

Diagnoses A is tiered as **clinically high** likelihood. The disease explains all the patient's major findings. The patient has all significant manifestations of the disease. The patient has no major rejecting features and has a key feature. In this tier, a very likely diagnosis has a pre-test probability of more than 90% if the patient has a key feature of the disease. A likely diagnosis usually has a pre-test probability of 67% to 90%; there are no major rejecting features and no key feature.

Diagnoses B is tiered as **clinically moderate** likelihood. The disease explains most of the patient's major findings. The patient lacks some of the usual features of the disease. They are no rejecting features. In this tier, the pre-test probability of the diagnosis is about 34% to 66%.

Diagnoses C is tiered as **clinically low** likelihood. The patient has single or few features of the disease in question. The patient has a rejecting feature of the disease in question. In this tier, the pre-test probability of the diagnosis is less than 33%. The diagnosis is very unlikely if the diagnosis is less than 10% pre-test probability; this usually means a **rejecting feature t**hat makes the diagnosis very unlikely.

The compare and contrast method are used in the analysis of diagnosis A, B, and C. As seen in Figure 7, the syndrome diagnosis is the common feature found in all three diagnoses. There are three important components in the differential diagnoses: Key Feature, Differentiating Feature, and Rejecting Feature. The **key feature** is the most striking clinical feature, making it the most likely clinical symptom or sign that clinches the diagnosis. The **differentiating feature** is a major feature common with two diagnoses but not present in the other diagnosis. This means Diagnosis A and B have a common differentiating feature that is not found in Diagnosis C. Diagnosis A and C have a common differentiating feature that is not found in Diagnosis B. Diagnoses B and C have a common differentiating feature that is not found in Diagnosis A. Identifying the key and differentiating features are essential in the proper selection of the differential diagnoses. Diagnoses C usually contains rejecting features, the absence or presence of a clinical symptom or sign that makes the diagnoses the least likely cause of the patient's illness.

There are different combinations of the diagnostic triad based on the pre-test probability of the diagnoses. Sometimes, there may be no clinically high probability diagnoses because the signs and symptoms, disease pathology, and localization are not well defined. In the ideal setting, we should have a combination of Diagnoses A, B, C. Other diagnostic triad possibilities are:

Diagnoses A, B, B: There is a diagnosis with a very high pre-test probability but with two other diagnoses with moderate likelihood pre-test probability. A key feature is present in one of the diagnostic triads. The latter have no rejecting features. A confirmatory diagnostic test or procedure may be needed to rule in Diagnosis A or rule out Diagnoses B.

Diagnoses B, B, B: All three diagnoses have moderate likelihood pre-test probability for the diagnoses. There is no key feature among the choices. In this scenario, the syndrome has many diseases where the signs and symptoms are closely related. This can be seen in genetic disorders where the phenotype features are closely similar. Hence, a highly specific or sensitive diagnostic test is needed to rule in or rule out disease, respectively.

Diagnoses, B, B, C: Two diagnoses have a moderate likelihood pre-test probability but no key feature that stands out. The third differential diagnoses have a low pre-test likelihood probability as the primary diagnosis.

Diagnoses B, C, C: In this situation, the clinical information may not have sufficient data, and only one differential diagnosis may have a moderate degree of pre-test probability. The other two differential diagnoses may have a few features and signs but with a low pre-test probability.

Case Study:

E.D. is a 65-year-old male who was admitted for confusion. About eight weeks ago, he was waking up disoriented. He reported seeing shadows in his room. About seven weeks ago, he started falling and clumsy when he walks. He was sometimes clumsy with his right hand. Six weeks before his admission, he was becoming more forgetful and got startled easily. He gradually started to decline in his self-care, dressing, bathing and eating. He was becoming quiet and withdrawn. He was having involuntary movements of the limbs. There is no family history of dementia, suicide, or seizures. He is a retired policeman. He does not smoke or drink alcohol. He has no record of head trauma, fever,

Illness Script: E.D. is a 65-year-old male with a rapidly progressive cognitive decline associated with bilateral limb ataxia, generalized myoclonus, bilateral cogwheel rigidity, wide-based gait, and unsteadiness. The localization indicates diffuse involvement of the cerebral cortex, basal ganglia, and cerebellar regions of the CNS.

Disease Syndrome Script: E. D. is a 65-year-old male with a rapidly progressive cognitive decline associated with bilateral limb ataxia, generalized myoclonus, bilateral cogwheel rigidity, wide-based gait, and unsteadiness. The clinical features are consistent with dementia, parkinsonism, and pan-cerebellar syndrome, which indicates a diffuse involvement of the cerebral cortex, basal ganglia, and cerebellar regions of the CNS.

Disease Script: E.D. is an elderly 65-year-old male with subacute, rapidly progressive cognitive decline, bilateral limb ataxia, generalized myoclonus, bilateral cogwheel rigidity, wide-based gait, and unsteadiness. The clinic features are consistent with progressive dementia, parkinsonism, and pan-cerebellar syndrome. The disease mechanism may be toxic, autoimmune, infectious, or neoplastic disease pathology.

Diagnostic Triad:

Diagnosis A: Creutzfeldt-Jakob (CJD): The key feature is the rapidly progressive dementia and myoclonus.

Diagnosis B: Lewy Body Disease (LBD): CJD and LBD can present with Dementia and Parkinsonism. The course is usually gradual and associated with visual hallucinations.

Diagnosis C: Alzheimer's Disease (AD): Gradual cognitive decline is a common feature of AD; however, the course is not rapid. Parkinsonism and Cerebellar signs are not common with AD.

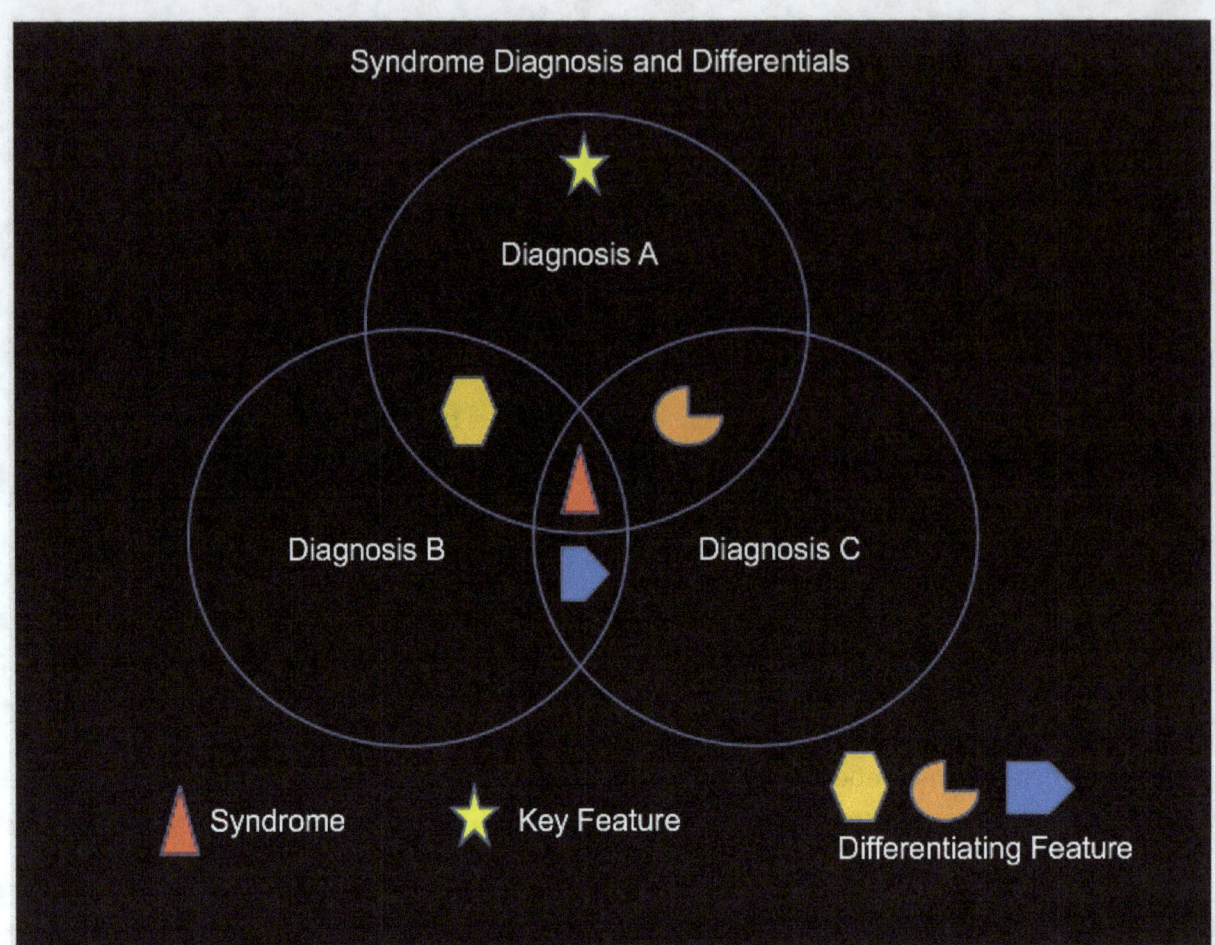

Figure 7. Syndrome Diagnoses and Differential Diagnoses. The Key Feature (star) is the most striking clinical feature, making it the most likely clinical symptom or sign that clinches the diagnoses. The differentiating feature is a major feature found common with 2 of the diagnoses but not present in the other diagnosis. Diagnosis A and B have a common differentiating feature not found in Diagnosis C. Diagnosis A and C have a common differentiating feature not found in Diagnosis B. Diagnoses B and C have a common differentiating feature not found in Diagnosis A.

CLINICAL ASSESSMENT AND RECOMMENDATIONS (CARE)

After formulating the differential diagnoses, the clinician should construct the assessment and plan of care. There are four parts to this medical documentation. The first part is the neurological summary. The second part will be the diagnosis, and the third, the plan of care. The fourth part is the outcome and prognosis.

I. Neurological Summary:

This would be the concise description of the neurological history, objective findings, and neurological localization **(patient illness script).** The physician should summarize in 3 sentences (at minimum) the clinical history, physical findings, and neurological localization. The first sentence is the clinical history. The second sentence is the salient findings. The salient results can include laboratory or radiographic data if present. In the initial encounter, the laboratory data or imaging may not be available. Hence, the pertinent physical and neurological findings should only be cited. The third sentence is neurological localization. *If there are additional supporting data, the patient disease syndrome or disease script can be incorporated in the summary.*

Example 1: Neurologic Summary (Initial encounter):

Mr. Brown is a 55-year-old male, admitted for sudden/acute right-sided weakness and speech impairment. The pertinent findings are BP of 220/100, irregular heart rhythm, obesity, right face, arm and leg weakness, and global aphasia. The localization is the left frontal-parietal cortical region.

Example 2: Neurologic Summary (Progress notes):

Mr. Brown is a 55-year-old male and admitted for sudden right hemiplegia and speech impairment. On the 2nd hospital day, the pertinent findings showed a reduction of his blood pressure to 140/90, atrial fibrillation, complete right hemiplegia, global aphasia, a cardiac ejection fraction of 20%, left hemisphere PLEDs (EEG), and left frontal and parietal diffusion-weighted imaging signal abnormalities (MRI). The clinical, EEG, and radiographic localization is consistent with a lesion involving the left middle cerebral artery distribution.

After the neurological summary, the physician will compose the diagnosis. This consists of 4 domains or categories.

A. Diagnosis: Syndrome, Disease, or Symptom-based:

It is customary in the neurological diagnosis to localize the signs and symptoms and incorporate a syndromic diagnosis **(patient disease syndrome script).** A syndrome is a set of signs and symptoms. The neurologist formulates a hypothesis on the syndrome for the patient. A neurological syndrome may be generic syndrome for a group of diseases, i.e., Parkinsonism.

Once further workup reveals the underlying or specific disease, the neurologist can be precise and disease-specific, i.e., Acute Ischemic Stroke, Left Middle Cerebral Artery distribution (**patient disease script**). If the syndrome diagnosis or disease-specific diagnosis cannot be made, a symptom-based approach will be the alternative, i.e., Acute Headache.

B. Etiology:

If disease-specific diagnosis is made, an etiology can usually be categorized. The specific etiology for the disease should be clearly written in this domain. For example, carotid dissection. However, there are different causes or etiologies to a neurological syndrome or disease. If the diagnosis is symptom-based, the etiology is usually unknown. When unknown or multiple causes, the top considerations or differential etiologies are placed in parenthesis. If the clinician only has syndrome diagnosis, it would be an excellent exercise to have three differential diagnoses **(diagnostic triad)** stated in this domain.

C. Functional impairment:

Functional impairment is a vital assessment category. Often, referring physicians, physical/speech/occupational therapists would like to know the physical impairment. In following the clinical course of a patient, the functional impairment may improve or worsen. This will become relevant when different providers are reviewing the clinical course of the patient. It will also help the physician know if the intervention was effective or not. Importantly, insurance providers often request medical records of the patient when a disability application is made.

D. Related Condition/Risk/Co-Morbidity

The fourth domain identifies conditions, risk factors, or comorbidities contributing to the patient's present neurological condition. This may also serve as the secondary diagnosis.

The recommendations are composed of 2 domains or categories:

(1) Diagnostic Recommendations:

The recommendations should list in importance the test that would support the diagnosis and list other tests that are needed to rule out other disease entities.

(2) Therapeutic Recommendations:

The therapeutic recommendations are the treatment interventions in priority order for a specific patient.

Example:

Plan of Care:

Diagnostic: MRI brain, Carotid Ultrasound, Echocardiogram, Lipid Profile, Serum Chemistries, PT/PTT/INR, CBC

Therapeutic: Oral Coumadin 5-10 mg per day. DVT prophylaxis, PT/OT/Speech therapy, Stroke Education, Smoking Cessation

Prognosis and Outcome:

Each patient will need serial assessments on the response to treatment (outcome) and prognosis of the underlying neurological disease. In the initial encounter, this may be undetermined because diagnosis procedures are still done, and treatment may be in the early stages. On subsequent inpatient follow-up or clinic visits/progress notes, the physician can comment on the patient's outcome from the treatment or intervention (if any). Patients, family members, and referring physicians are often interested in the neurological condition's course or prognosis.

Example:

On day five post-stroke, the INR is now 2.3. The anticoagulation goal is between 2-3. Blood pressure is controlled and is currently 120/70. The severity of his stroke suggests a poor prognosis for full functional recovery.

Case Illustration:

DL is a 25-year-old right-handed male. He was referred for a headache evaluation. He has chronic daily headaches for the past five months. The headache was holocranial and pounding. It was persistent, and it waxed and waned. He had three severe headaches per week. He has no nausea or light sensitivity. Physical activity or lying down made the headache worse. In the last four weeks, he had horizontal diplopia. He has not been able to drive because of diplopia. He has no change in his walking or bladder functions. He has no limb weakness or incoordination. He has no change in his speech, memory, behavior, or personality. Swallowing and articulation were not affected. He has no known medical problems except for obesity. He takes anti-acne medication for the past 12 months. The general examination is normal, with a Body Mass Index of 32. The pertinent neurological findings showed bilateral optic disc swelling and abduction weakness of lateral gaze towards the right or left. The upgaze and downgaze were normal

Clinical Assessment and Recommendation (CARE):

Neurological Summary: DL is a 25-year-old male with chronic daily headache and diplopia for five months in the context of daily intake of anti-acne medication. He has obesity, bilateral papilledema, and bilateral abduction weakness of the eyes. The localization is diffuse, affecting probably the meningeal, sinus-venous, arterial, or spinal fluid circulation of the cerebrum, both optic nerves (cranial nerve II) and abducens nerve (cranial nerve VI). He has secondary chronic headache syndrome. The disease mechanism may be iatrogenic (drugs), inflammatory, infectious, vascular, neoplastic, or endocrine. *Comment: the neurological summary is the patient disease script.*

Neurological Diagnosis: The chronic headache syndrome differential diagnoses are benign intracranial hypertension (iatrogenic/drug), chronic meningitis (infectious), or chronic sinus-venous thrombosis (vascular). *Comment: the neurological diagnosis is the patient's diagnostic triad.*

Etiology: Probably drug-induced from anti-acne medication

Functional Impairment: visual impairment from diplopia

Related Condition: Obesity is related to intracranial hypertension.

Recommendations:

Diagnostic:

CT scan brain without contrast today

Lumbar puncture if CT scan brain is normal. Check opening pressure. CSF routine studies and culture.

Schedule for MRI brain with and without contrast/ MR venography

ESR, TSH, CMP, CBC, Platelet count, PT

Therapeutic:

Pending; it depends on the CT scan result today.

Outcome and Prognosis: pending.

Follow Up Visit #1:

   DL had his CT scan of the head on the day of the clinic visit. He returned the following day after being informed that the head's CT showed no midline shifts or mass. He consented to the lumbar puncture procedure. The opening pressure was 35 cm water (lateral decubitus), and 15 ml of CSF was drained. The closing pressure was 12 cm water. He had dramatic relief from his headache and double vision. CSF studies showed no WBC, normal protein, and glucose. The gram stain of CSF was negative. The CSF cultures were pending. CBC, platelet, TSH, CMP were normal. The MRI brain with MR venography was not yet done and was scheduled for the following week. The patient was informed to discontinue his anti-acne medication.

CARE Follow Up Visit #1

Neurological Summary: DL is a 25-year-old male with chronic daily headache and diplopia for five months in the context of daily intake of anti-acne medication. He has obesity, bilateral papilledema, and bilateral abduction weakness of the eyes. The localization was diffuse, affecting sinus-venous cerebrospinal fluid circulation in the cerebrum. This manifested as optic disc nerve swelling/papilledema (cranial nerve II) and abducens nerve palsy (cranial nerve VI). He has chronic headache syndrome secondary to elevated intracranial pressure. The CT head, CBC, CMP, TSH, ESR were normal. The high CSF pressure confirmed intracranial hypertension. The CSF studies were normal. The disease mechanism is likely iatrogenic from anti-acne medication.

Neurological Diagnosis: Benign Intracranial Hypertension

Etiology: Drug-induced from anti-acne medication

Functional Impairment: visual impairment from diplopia

Related Condition: Obesity

Recommendations:

Diagnostic:

Proceed MRI brain with and without contrast/ MR venography to exclude sinus-venous thrombosis.

Therapeutic:

Stopping the anti-acne medication

Acetazolamide 250 mg twice a day for four weeks.

Counseling on weight loss

Outcome and Prognosis: the patient had an excellent response with CSF drainage. The prognosis is usually when the offending agent is discontinued.

Follow Up Visit #2

DL is asymptomatic since he started the Acetazolamide 250 mg twice a day, and he has stopped taking the anti-acne medication for the last four weeks. He was able to drive and did not experience any double vision. He lost 10 pounds since his previous visit. MR venography done three weeks ago was normal. The MRI brain with and without contrast was normal. Neurological examination showed no papilledema. He had normal pursuit and saccadic eye movements.

CARE Follow up Visit #2

Neurological Summary: DL is a 25-year-old male with chronic daily headache and diplopia for five months in the context of daily intake of anti-acne medication. He has obesity, bilateral papilledema, and bilateral abduction weakness of the eyes. The localization was diffuse, affecting sinus-venous cerebrospinal fluid circulation in the cerebrum. This manifested as optic disc papilledema (cranial nerve II) and abducens nerve palsy (cranial nerve VI). He has chronic headache syndrome secondary to elevated intracranial pressure. The CT head, CBC, CMP, TSH, and ESR were normal. The high CSF pressure confirmed intracranial hypertension. The CSF studies were normal. The disease mechanism was iatrogenic (medication intake). This was confirmed when the papilledema and headache resolved after the anti-acne medication was stopped.

Neurological Diagnosis: Benign Intracranial Hypertension

Etiology: Drug-induced/Anti-acne medication

Functional Impairment: none; diplopia resolved

Related Condition: Obesity is related to intracranial hypertension.

Recommendations:

Diagnostic: None

Therapeutic: Discontinue Diamox. Observe for headache recurrence.

Outcome/Prognosis: With the offending agent removed, the prognosis is excellent. With the Diamox discontinued, we can assess if the patient is in complete remission.

Appendix I

Instruments for Neurological Examination

Reflex Hammer :

There are different types of a reflex hammers. They are used to elicit deep tendon reflexes (muscle stretch reflexes and percussion myotonia). The reflex Hammer shown is the Babinski Hammer, Taylor Hammer, Tromner Hammer, and Buck reflex Hammer from left to right.

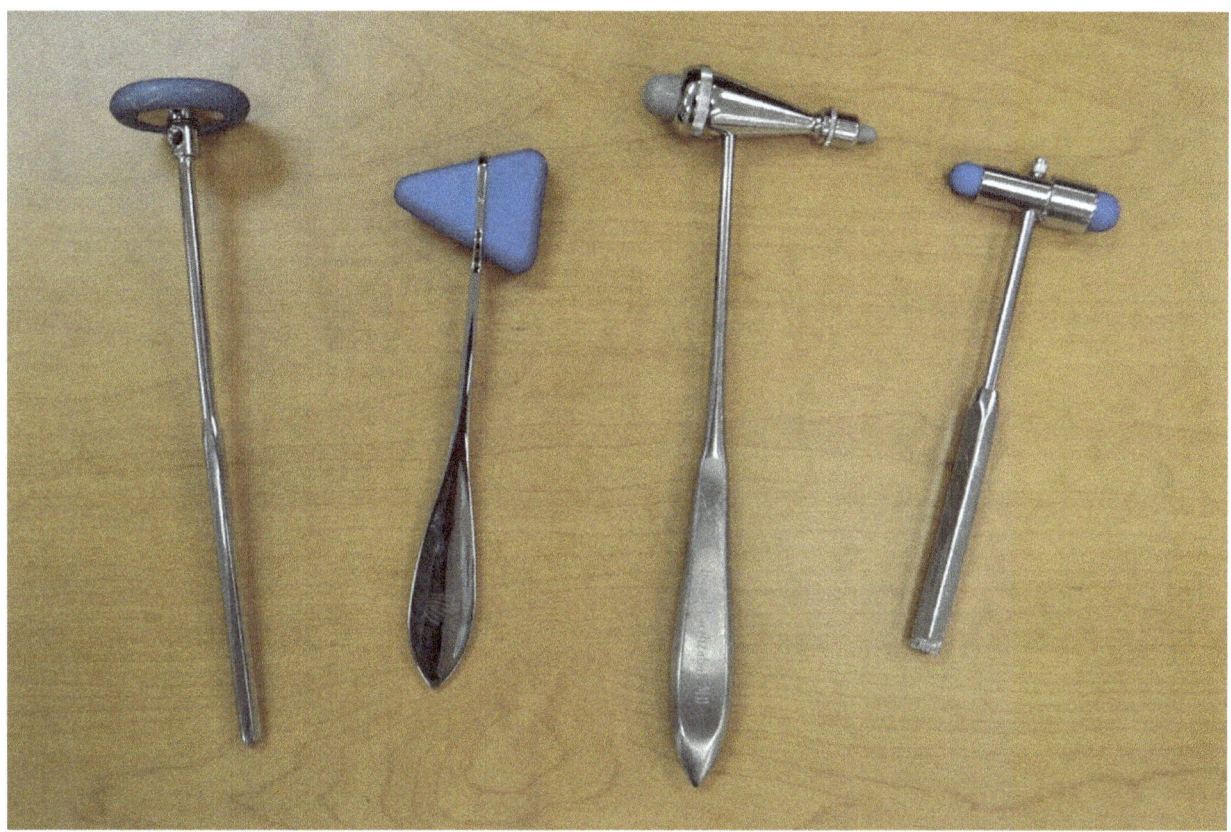

Pin

The pin is used for pain perception. An unused safety pin can be a substitute. The pin is used to test the pain perception of the limb and body. It can help demarcate the type of sensory deficit (nerve root, peripheral nerve, or dermatomal). It may also be used to test pain perception of the head and face for individuals having significant sensory deficits.

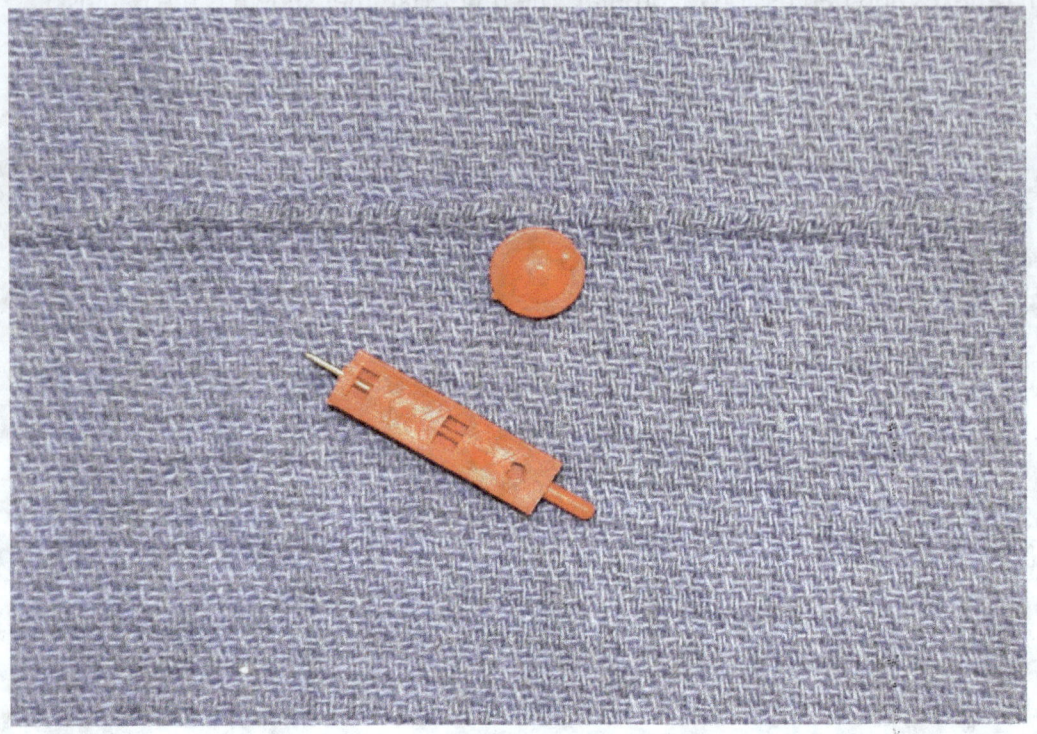

Cotton

The cotton swab stick or wisp of cotton is used for light touch sensory testing of the face and limbs. Clean cotton is also used to test the corneal sensation and the corneal reflex.

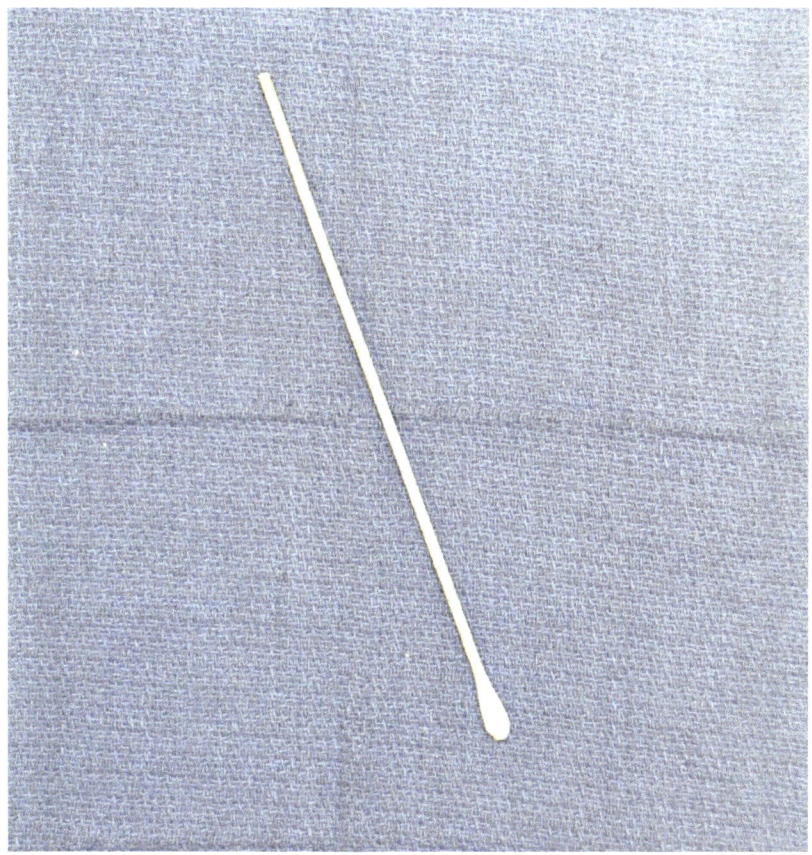

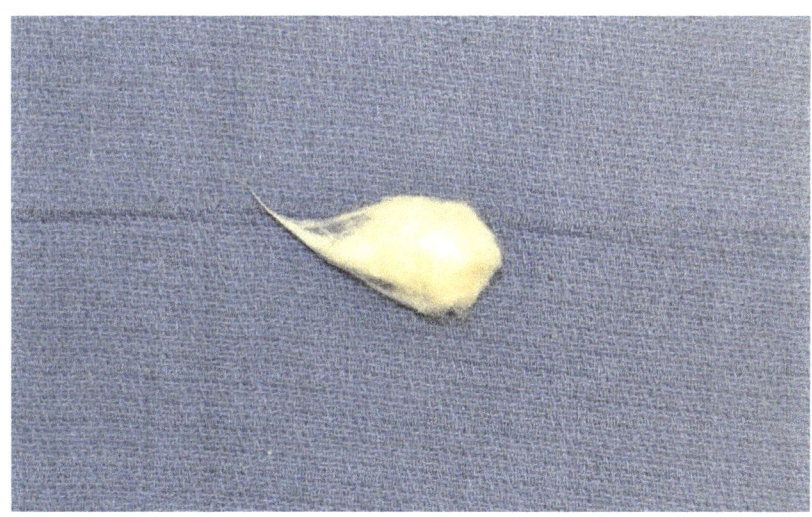

Tuning Fork

There are different types of tuning fork. It resonates at different frequencies. The left fork resonates at 128 Hz and is used for vibration perception of the distal limbs. The right fork resonates at 256 Hz and is used for Weber's and Rinne's auditory testing.

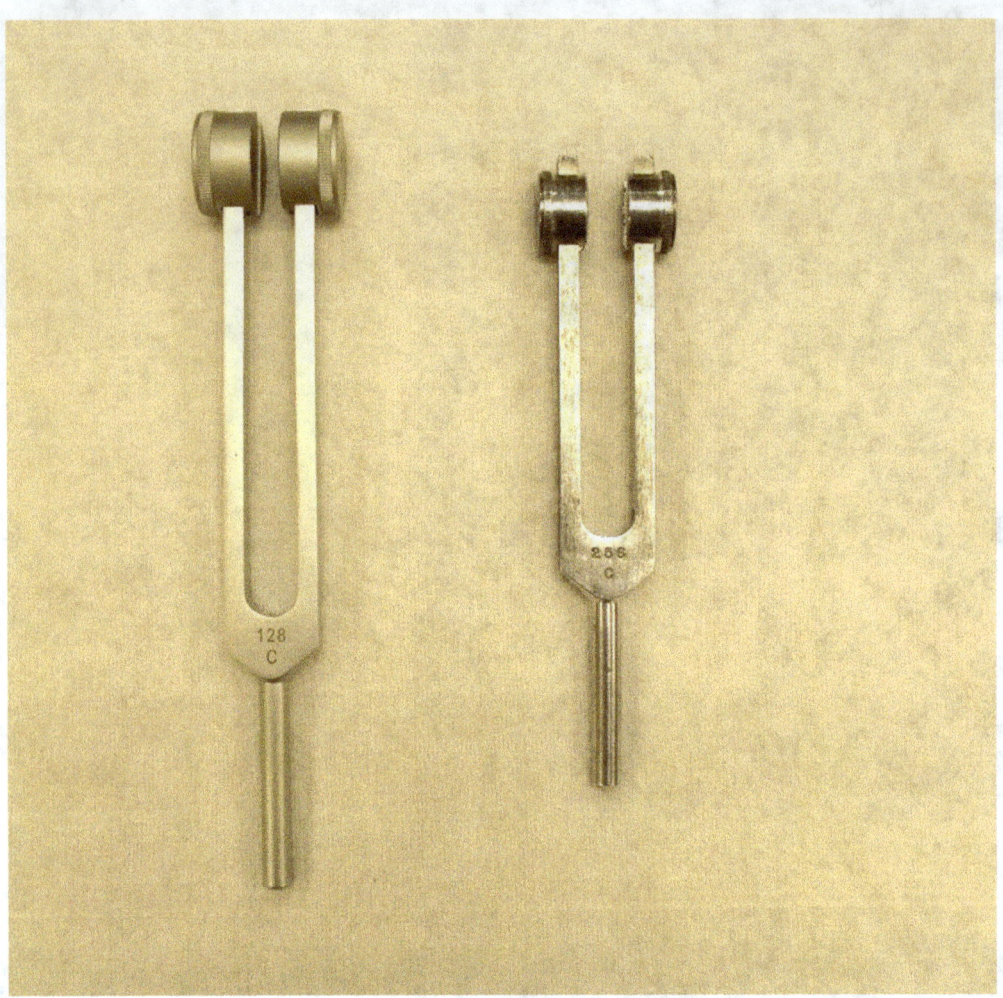

Two-point discriminator

The instrument below is for discriminatory sensory testing, and it measures the minimum distance that a person can identify between two points. The minimum distance perception varies on the body part tested. The fingers and tongue are more sensitive to identify two distinct points. In contrast, sensory perception of 2 points of the back has a broader distance for 2 point discrimination.

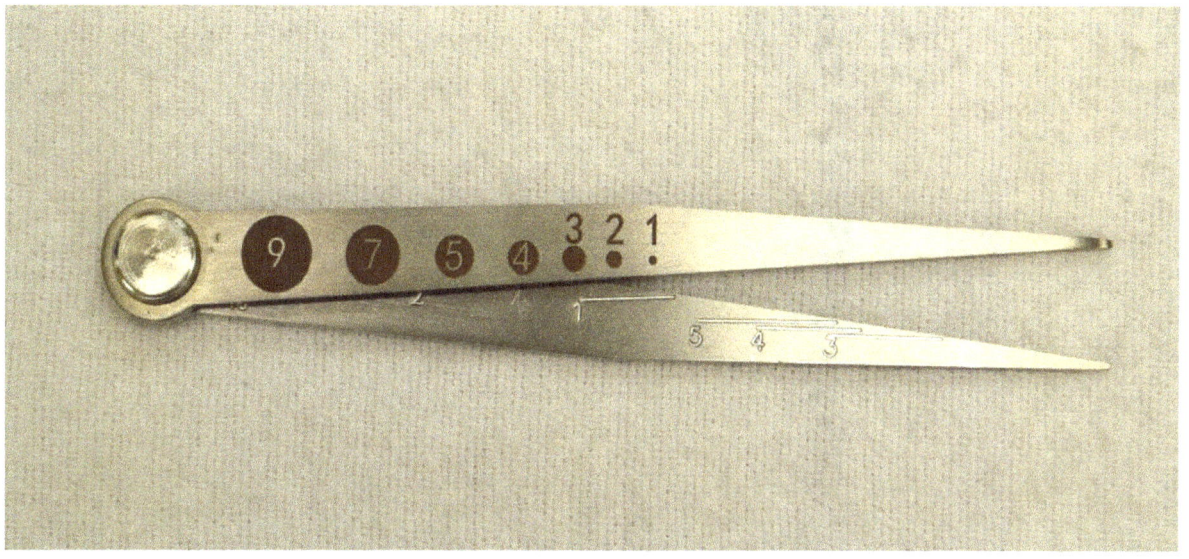

Eye Cover/Occluder

During confrontation eye testing, the left or right eye is tested individually. The patient may use the eye cover/occluder to cover one eye. If not available, the patient can cover their eye with their hand.

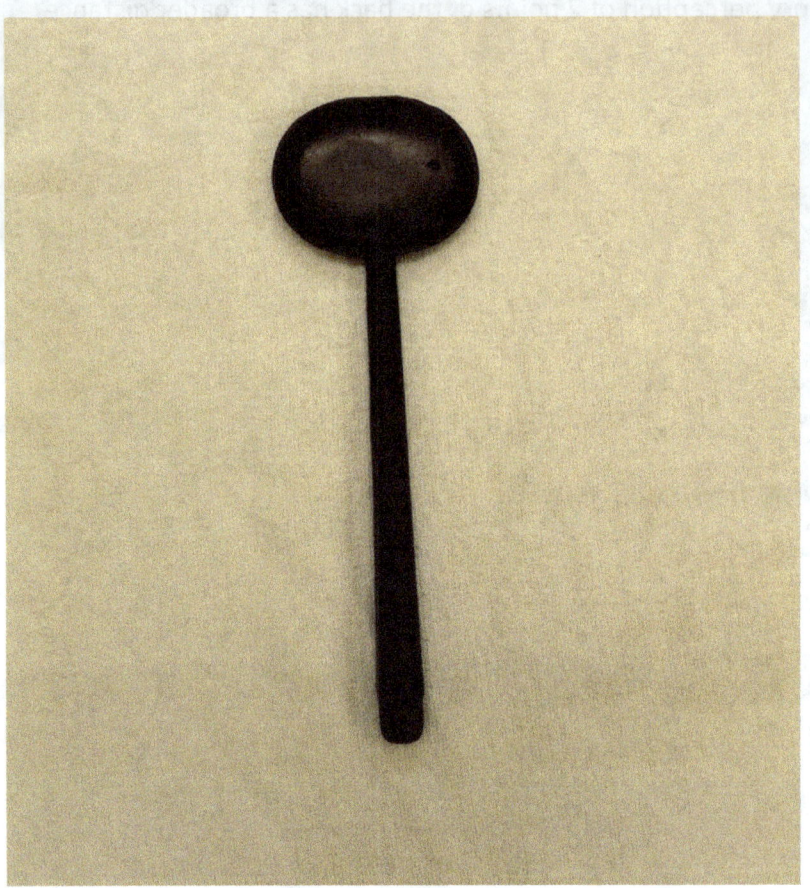

Penlight

The penlight is used to test pupil reaction and examination of the posterior pharynx during gag testing.

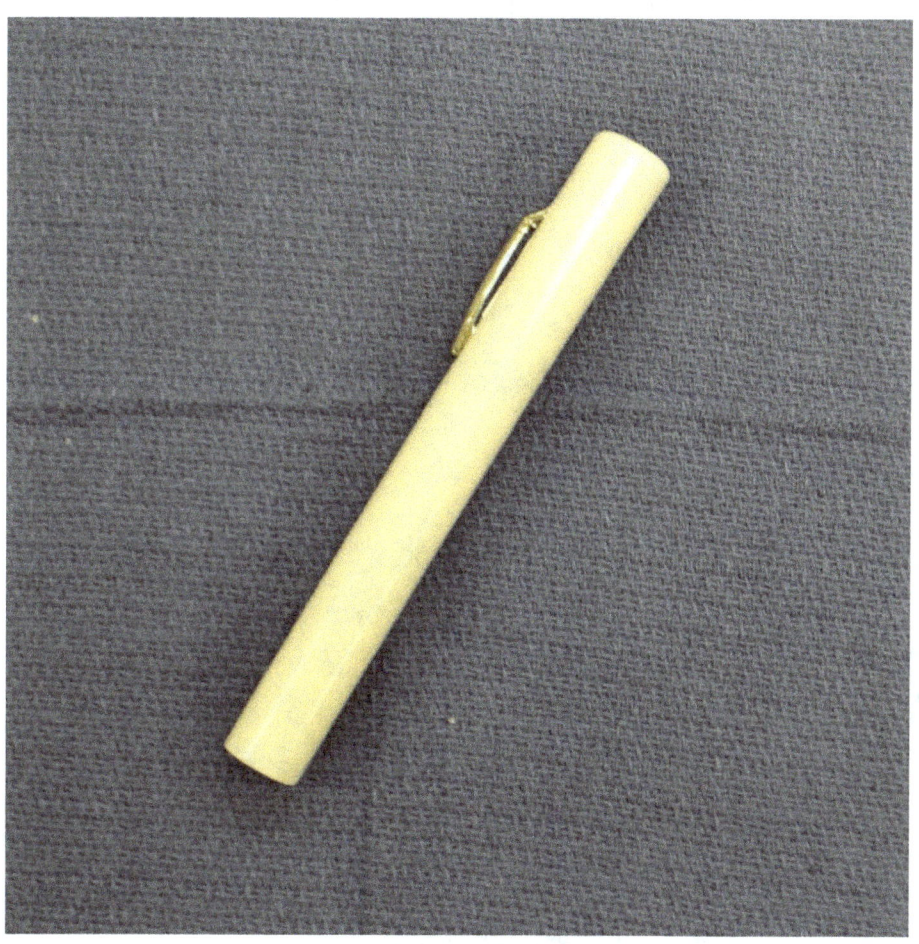

Ophthalmoscope and Otoscope

An ophthalmoscope is used to examine the optic disc and retina. For patients with headaches, checking the optic disc for edema or papilledema is mandatory. It is also used to check for hypertensive or diabetic retinopathy. The otoscope is used for examining the auditory canal and eardrum. Otoscopy is an essential examination for patients with hearing impairment before doing a Weber and Rinne testing.

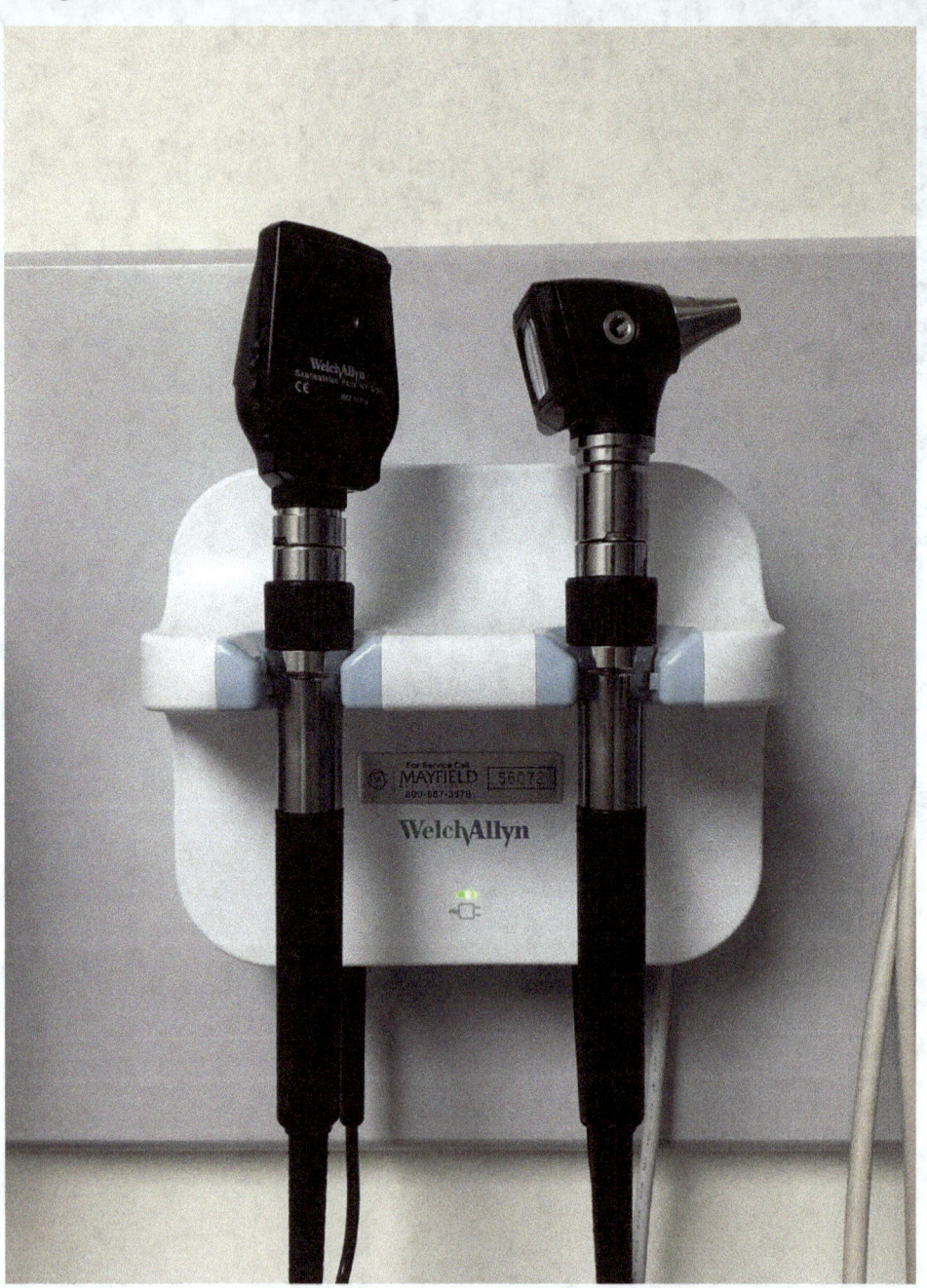

Optic Nerve Card

A pocket visual card to check near-vision or visual acuity is an essential test for in cranial nerve II (optic nerve)

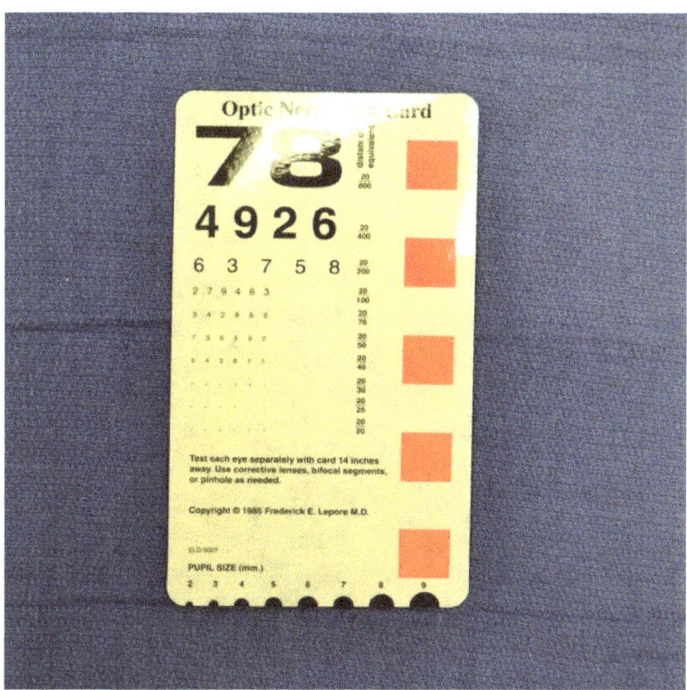

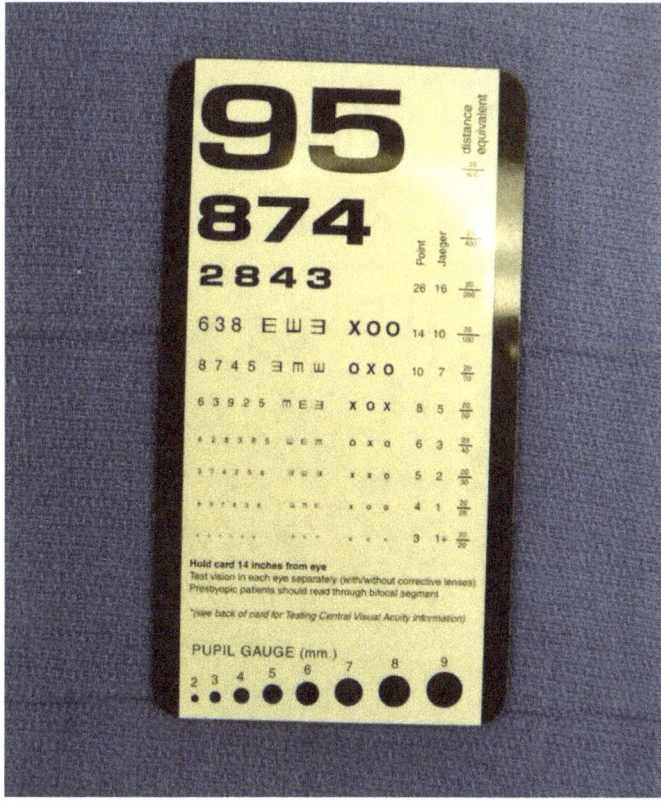

Tongue Blade

The tongue blade is used to examine the posterior pharynx and to elicit the gag reflex.

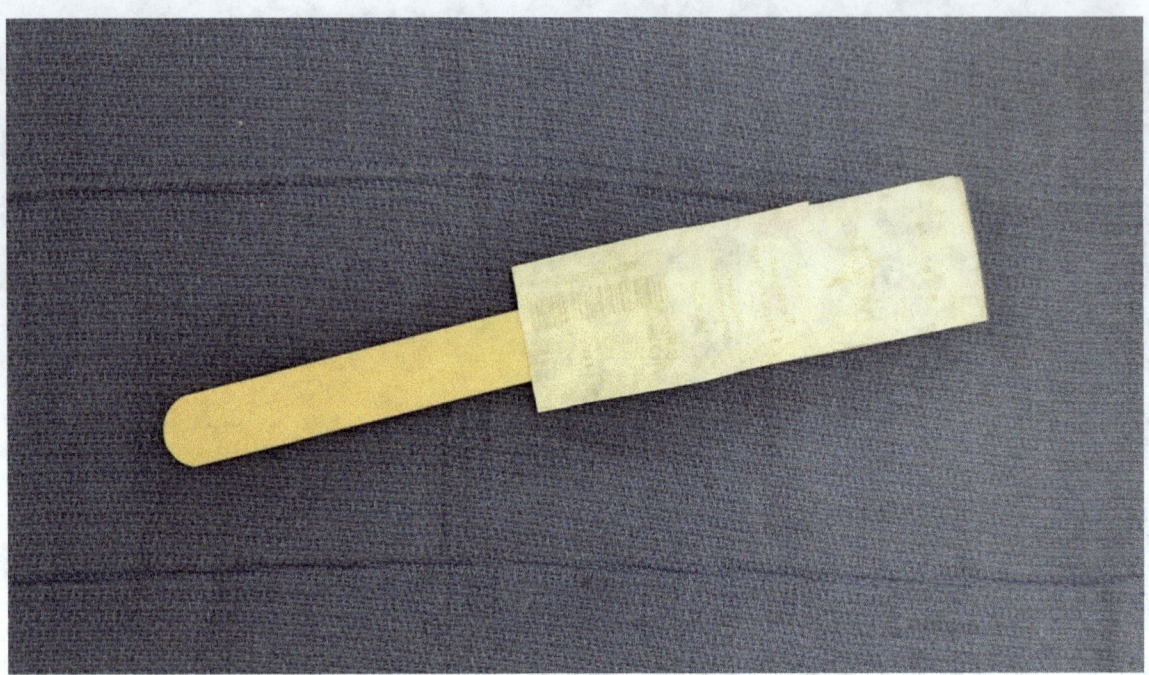

Appendix II

Functional Anatomy of Neurological Categories

Neurological Category	Anatomical Structures
Consciousness	Cerebral Hemisphere, Upper Brainstem
Sleep	Hypothalamus
	Brainstem
Cognition	Cerebral Cortex
Behavior and Mood	Temporal Lobe, Limbic Lobe
Thought Content	Frontal, Temporal, Parietal Lobe
Neuroendocrine	Hypothalamus
	Pituitary gland
Special Senses	
Vision	Retina, optic nerve, optic radiation, visual cortex
Smell	Olfactory nerve, Olfactory bulb, Olfactory Tract
	Olfactory Cortex (Piriformis, Amygdala, Entorhinal cortex)
	Orbitofrontal Cortex
Auditory	Auditory nerve, brainstem, temporal lobe
Brainstem/Cranial Nerves	Midbrain, CN III, IV
	Pons, CN V, VI, VII, VIII
	Medulla, CN IX, X, XI, XII
Primary Motor System	Primary motor cortex
	Internal capsule, posterior limb
	Brainstem
	Spinal Cord, Anterior horn
Secondary Motor System	Basal ganglia
	Cerebellum
	Brainstem, Spinal Cord
Primary and Discriminatory Sensation	Parietal cortex, Thalamus, Spinothalmaic tract, and posterior column of spinal cord
Autonomics	Parasympathetic Nervous System
	Brainstem – cranial nerves III, V, IX, X
	Spinal Cord – Sacral S2-S4
	Sympathetic Nervous System
	Spinal Cord – Thoracic, Lumbar

www.ingramcontent.com/pod-product-compliance
Lightning Source LLC
Chambersburg PA
CBHW081454220526
45466CB00008B/2645